Getting into

Medical School

2019 Entry

Getting into guides

Getting into Art & Design Courses, 10th edition

Getting into Business & Economics Courses, 12th edition

Getting into Dental School, 10th edition

Getting into Engineering Courses, 4th edition

Getting into Law, 12th edition

Getting into Medical School 2019 Entry, 23rd edition

Getting into Oxford & Cambridge 2019 Entry, 21st edition

Getting into Pharmacy and Pharmacology Courses, 2nd edition

Getting into Physiotherapy Courses, 9th edition

Getting into Psychology Courses, 12th edition

Getting into Veterinary School, 11th edition

How to Complete Your UCAS Application 2019 Entry, 30th edition

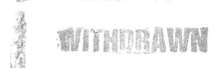
Getting into

Medical School

2019 Entry

James Barton and
Simon Horner

23rd edition

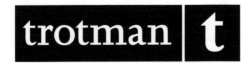

Getting into Medical School

This 23rd edition published in 2018 by Trotman Education, an imprint of Crimson Publishing Ltd, 21d Charles Street, Bath BA1 1HX

© Crimson Publishing Ltd 2018

Authors: James Barton and Simon Horner
15th edn: Simon Horner and Steven Piumatti
16th–17th edns: Simon Horner
18th–22nd edns: James Barton and Simon Horner

British Library Cataloguing in Publication Data
A catalogue record for this book is available from the British Library

ISBN 978 1 911067 82 5

Printed and bound in the UK by 4edge Limited

Contents

Contents

About the authors

James Barton is Director of Admissions at Mander Portman Woodward's London college, and has worked there since September 2007. As well as being the author of *Getting into Veterinary School* and *Getting into Physiotherapy Courses*, James has sat on interview and audition panels and has given careers advice, talks and public seminars across a range of fields, both domestically and internationally. This is his sixteenth Trotman publication.

Simon Horner is Head of Science at Mander Portman Woodward in London and co-runs the college's medical programme, which includes lectures, seminars and mock interview practice for both internal and external students. This is Simon's sixth Trotman publication.

Acknowledgements

In order to write this book, we have needed help from many sources. Without the help of the medical schools' admissions departments, this book would not exist, and we would like to record our gratitude to all of the people who gave up their time to answer our questions. Thanks here to Max Butler, Robert Miller, Jess Polkey, Freddie Champion, Lucy Dunn, Connor Jenkins, Arthur Knowles and Tara Bage, who are currently embarking on what will no doubt be successful medical careers. A special thank you also goes to Kal Makwana for his valuable consultancy throughout the research. MediPathways is an excellent initiative and one we believe will continue to go from strength to strength under Kal's stewardship. We would also like to say thank you to UCAS, who provided us with the data we required, and to Della Oliver and Emma Davies for the help they provided in producing this book.

We would like to dedicate this book to Mr John Horner.

James Barton and Simon Horner
November 2017

About this book

First of all, a note on terminology. Throughout this guide, the term 'medical school' includes the university departments of medicine. Second, entry requirements have been quoted in A level terms; a general guide to the grades or scores that you need if you are taking Scottish Highers, the International Baccalaureate or other qualifications can be found on pages 2–3.

This book is divided into nine main chapters, which aim to cover three major obstacles that would-be doctors may face:

* getting an interview at medical school
* getting a conditional offer
* getting the right A level grades (or equivalent).

The nine chapters discuss the following:

1. the study of medicine
2. the application process and getting an interview
3. the interview process
4. current issues that may come up at interview
5. results day
6. non-standard applications
7. fees and funding
8. careers opportunities
9. further information.

Chapter 1 gives information on the actual study of medicine, different teaching styles and postgraduate study as well as possible specialisations and post-degree course options.

Chapter 2 deals with the preparation that you will need to undertake in order to make your application as irresistible as possible to get an offer and/or an interview. It includes advice on work experience, how to choose a medical school, sample questions from admissions tests such as UKCAT and BMAT and the mechanics of the UCAS application process.

Chapter 3 provides advice on what to expect at the interview stage, current topics, issues you may be questioned on and how to ensure that you come across as a potential doctor.

Chapter 4 presents some key information on contemporary and topical medical issues, such as the structure of the NHS, world health and statistics on some of the most well-known diseases and illnesses.

Knowing about medical issues is a must, particularly if you are called in for an interview.

Chapter 5 looks at the options that you have at your disposal on results day and describes the steps that you need to take if you are holding an offer or if you have been unsuccessful and have not been given an offer.

Chapter 6 is aimed primarily at overseas students and any other 'non-standard' applicants – mature students, graduates, students who have studied arts A levels and retake students (most medical schools consider non-standard applicants). The chapter also includes some advice for those who want to study medicine outside the UK, say, for example, in the US.

Chapter 7 gives some useful information regarding fees and funding for medical students, as well as bursaries and scholarships that are available, while **Chapter 8** looks at career options in medicine.

Finally, in **Chapter 9**, further information is given in terms of courses and further reading. A number of other excellent books are available on the subject of getting into medical school. The contact details of the various medical groups and universities can also be found here. After Chapter 9 a **glossary** can be found of many of the terms used throughout the book.

The difference between other guides on getting into medical school and this one is that this guide is a route map; it tells you the path to follow if you want to be a doctor. Because of this, it is rather bossy and dictatorial. We make no apology for this, because we have seen far too many aspiring medical students who took the wrong subjects, who didn't bother to find work experience and who never asked themselves why they wanted to be a doctor before their interviews. Their path into medicine was made unnecessarily difficult because they didn't prepare properly.

Throughout the book you will find case studies and examples of material that will reflect to some extent the theme being discussed at that point. We hope that you find these real-life examples illuminating.

Finally, the views expressed in this book, though informed by conversations with staff at medical schools and elsewhere, are our own, unless specifically attributed to a contributor in the text.

Is there a doctor in the house?
Introduction

'I always found science interesting and like the fact that I continue to learn on a daily basis, from books, journals and patients. I like the investigative challenge and nature of the job. General Practice is the opportunity to get to understand different patients and their needs, and it can be incredibly rewarding to take someone through their life cycle.'

Dr Vicki Cooney

In recent times, you cannot go through a day without hearing about the NHS. It is the media soft toy, often vilified, rarely championed and yet the reality is, the system is simply a victim of its own success. Yes, it is under-funded and frequently maligned in budgets. However, in the past 50 years, it has made enormous strides; and, on the eve of its 80th birthday, there is more than convincing reason to confidently argue that it is better now than ever. It has become better at saving people's lives. This is enormously positive and yet it means its failures become more transparent as public expectation in the healthcare sector is now at a level whereby they expect to be saved.

All that said, there are not enough doctors. That is where you come in. Or is it? This book is designed to show you how to get your place at medical school. With 1,500 extra places announced by the government for medical students in September 2018, as well as a pending review of the cap on the numbers universities can enrol on the course in the next few years, there has never been a better time to try and join the medical professions.

A realistic chance

Only around 40% of applicants for medicine are successful in gaining places. Does this mean that the remaining 60% were unsuitable? The answer, of course, is no. Many of those who are rejected are extremely strong candidates, with high grades at GCSE under their belts and the personalities and qualities that would make them into excellent doctors. There are a fixed number of medical school places available each year and so not all candidates can be successful. But many promising applicants do not put themselves in a position whereby they can be given proper consideration, simply because they do not prepare well enough.

Ideally, your preparation should begin at least two years before you submit your application, but if you have come to the decision to apply to study medicine more recently, or if you were unaware of what steps you need to take in order to prepare a strong application, don't worry. It is not too late. Even over a relatively short period of time (a few months) you can put together a convincing application.

According to the latest available statistics from UCAS on entries and applicants for the 2017–18 application cycle intake into medical schools, there was a further small decrease in the number of applicants compared with the 2016–17 numbers, and an increase in the number of places accepted. In the last report, UCAS had received 52,030 applications for medical school places from UK students and a further 16,625 applications from international and EU students. Therefore, in 2017–18, around 68,655 (down from 74,860 in the year before) students were battling for approximately 7,750 places available at UK medical schools.

UK students were more successful in gaining places (11.4% of applicants gained places) than international students, of whom only about 6% were successful and EU students, who had a 3% success rate. Female applicants outnumbered male applicants – 60% (up 1% on 2016–17) of all applicants were female – and success rates were slightly in favour of the female candidates.

Table 1 gives some comparisons and data on the 2017–2018 application cycle.

Table 1 Number of applicants in the 2017–18 academic year

Type of applicant	Number of applicants	Applicants accepted on to degree courses	Successful applicants (%)
UK	52,030	6,770	13.01
EU	5,885	255	4.33
Non-EU	10,740	725	6.75
Male	27,535	3,180	11.54
Female	41,120	4,570	11.11
Total	68,655	7,750	11.29

Source: www.ucas.com. We acknowledge UCAS' contribution of this information.

The grades you need

Table 12 (see pages 206–208) shows that, with a few exceptions, the A level grades you need for medicine are AAA, though there are some A* offers around now. You might be lucky and get an offer of AAB, but you won't know that until six months before the exams, so you can't rely on it. A number of medical schools, such as Cambridge, Oxford and Birmingham, are asking for an A* grade in their entry offers going forwards.

As a general guide, candidates with qualifications other than A levels are likely to need the following:

- Scottish: AAAAB in Highers or AA in Advanced Highers to include AAAAB in Highers
- International Baccalaureate: around 36–43 points, including 7, 6, 6 at Higher level (including chemistry)
- European Baccalaureate: roughly 80% overall, with at least 80% in chemistry and another full option science/mathematical subject.

But there's more to it than grades …

If getting a place to study medicine was purely a matter of achieving the right grades, medical schools would demand A*AA at A level (or equivalent) and 10 top grades at GCSE, and they would not bother to interview. However, to become a successful doctor requires many skills, academic and otherwise, and it is the job of the admissions staff to try to identify who of the thousands of applicants are the most suitable. It would be misleading to say that anyone, with enough effort, could become a doctor, but it is important for candidates who have the potential to succeed to make the best use of their applications.

Non-standard and second-time applications

Not all successful applicants apply during their final year of A levels. Some have retaken their exams, while others have used a gap year to add substance to their UCAS application. Again, it would be wrong to say that anyone who reapplies will automatically get a place, but good candidates should not assume that rejection first time round means the end of their medical career aspirations.

Gaining a place as a retake student or as a second-time applicant is not as easy as it used to be, but candidates who can demonstrate genuine commitment alongside the right personal and academic qualities still have a good chance of success if they go about their applications in the right way. The admissions staff at the medical schools tend to be extremely helpful and, except at the busiest times of the year when they simply do not have the time, they will give advice and encouragement to suitable applicants.

Admissions

The medical schools make strenuous efforts to maintain fair selection procedures: UCAS applications are generally seen by more than one selector, interview panels are given strict guidelines about what they can (and cannot) ask, and most make detailed statistics available about the backgrounds of the students they interview. Above all, admissions staff will tell you that they are looking for good 'all-rounders' who can communicate effectively with others, are academically able and are genuinely enthusiastic about medicine – if you think that this sounds like you, then read on!

Reflections of a doctor

The words below from a qualified practitioner and then from a final-year school student applying to study medicine express and reflect some of the many challenges and rewards that you may also face in your own journey to become a doctor. Like every journey, the grandest ones start with the first minuscule step.

The four stages/hurdles of doctordom

1 Deciding that it is what you want to do

Being called 'doctor' is pretty cool; it carries a certain social kudos and it's a big celebratory moment when your first piece of post arrives addressed to Dr instead of Ms or Mr. But is it for you? This decision is the first hurdle to clear, as it can be quite hard to step back and evaluate this for yourself once you have already started down the road to being a medical professional, so give it some thought now.

Aside from the pay, there are a great many advantages of being a doctor: it has great job security, a massive range of specialities and opportunities, allows you to perfect a variety of invaluable life skills, allows the opportunity to practise abroad and generally attracts a large number of people that make great lifelong friends.

However, it is important to think about some of the disadvantages and downsides of committing yourself to medicine. Whilst you imagine your life being synonymous to those starring on *Grey's Anatomy* or *Casualty*, medicine is hard work; no one – and I mean no one – gets through without pulling their finger out, and the work does not stop when you graduate; there are postgraduate exams and long, antisocial hours traipsing round a hospital surviving on boiled sweets the lovely lady recovering from her hip operation keeps offering you. You'll find that some patients believe that it is their right to have your constant attention and are as a result some-what less than friendly. In addition, whilst doctors have a great salary, you may find that friends from your maths and science classes at school begin to earn more by working in the City.

2 Getting into medical school

So you've decided to apply. Now you need to think what you can do that makes you stand out among the crowd of UK and interna-tional medical applicants. Is it the grade 8 didgeridoo or the 1,267 hours you spent working in a soup kitchen? Or do you, like most people, have to find new opportunities, skills and credentials for yourself to ensure that the admissions tutor does more than glance at your personal statement?

The advice I would give to those applying is:

- get as many people as possible to give feedback on your state-ment
- make sure you have adequate work experience (this doesn't need to be in a hospital; medical work is generally anything that involves looking after people)
- find someone to practise interviews with – it's very telling at interview who has thought about how to deal with difficult questions
- think carefully about where you are applying to and what makes the university different from others (every school thinks they are the best so it's worth bearing that in mind).

3 Passing medical school +/- intercalation

Finding how you work best is the key to medical school: are you a last-minute crammer, a lone worker, or a leader of a study group kind of person? If you can find out early, you can spend the whole of med school perfecting your own technique. In addition, it's important to continue all those extra-curricular activities that got you into medical school and try out new things once you get there. There's no such thing as not enough time to do things other than medicine – you're going to be busy for the rest of your life and managing your time is an important skill to learn as soon as you start.

4 Picking a specialty and future

Most people graduate from medical school around the age of 23 and by the time you get towards retirement you will probably have clocked at least 40 years in the working world. It is therefore important to think carefully about what your priorities are in life: flexible hours, promotion potential, minimising exams, working with children, or living in the countryside with four dogs and a pony. I suggest making a list now to see what you think you want. This will almost certainly change but it's worth learning to be reflective early on.

In conclusion, medicine is a fantastic career, and it is definitely a job for life. Think carefully about all the upcoming choices and good luck for the future.

Dr Sophie Lumley MBChB BMedSc
(healthcare ethics and law)
Academic FY1 doctor
Queen Elizabeth Hospital Birmingham

Case study

Arthur is in his final year of school and just embarking on his medical application. Here are his reflections on the process as it is ongoing.

'For the most part I was never completely sure what I wanted to do after school. I knew I had skills in certain subjects, especially biology, which I enjoyed. I had thought about medicine many times, but it wasn't until the first year of sixth form that my mind was made up.

'The first people I consulted about it were my friends and then my parents, who were all very supportive. I then began to look at universities to gain insight into the sorts of tests and the grades that I would need to have a chance at getting in.

'I attended a few lectures with my school, and at a Medlink conference at Nottingham University I met many other medicine applicants which reassured me of my chances as many were in the same boat as me.

'In the summer after my AS exams I had to take the UKCAT – UK Clinical Aptitude Test. Similar to an IQ test (it can be practised to increase scores), I was tested on mathematical, non-verbal and verbal reasoning skills, as well as my own situational judgement. My preparation for this test did not go as well as I would have hoped, but there are plenty of practice tests online to correct this.

'I left the booking of the test until quite late and got an earlier date for the test than I wanted. After having attended a festival I became ill before the day of the test which was at 8am! Apart from the first section – regrettably verbal reasoning – I did quite well in the test, which was a surprise. My advice to those taking the UKCAT would be to get an early insight into what the test is about and to practise a few questions, then, unlike me, you won't be anxious at the start. Furthermore, you should book the test as early as possible so that you can choose the best date to fit around your plans. Lastly, during the actual test, you should simply give it your best shot and not worry about not doing so well in a question or even a whole section, because this can easily be made up in the rest of the test. I don't think that most candidates answer all of the questions, due to time pressures and difficulties when spending too long on a single question.

'Work experience is also a major requirement, with each university specifying placements with direct patient care in a medical or non-medical environment. I did short amounts of work experience with various NHS services, such as an Emergency Response Team and a Sports Rehabilitation and Cardiac Clinic, as well as work experience in a care home. When I had a little more time, I got a placement in a ward of a small hospital, which allowed me to engage more with both patients and NHS staff which helped me to decide crucially whether or not I liked the idea of a medical role.

'The most important thing in my opinion when deciding whether or not to do medicine is if you truly have a passion for medical sciences and an underlying ambition to want to help those in need. Also, good communication skills and being ok with bodily fluids helps too.

'These factors can all be tested simply through engaging further with your subjects, talking to others, engaging with extra-curricular activities and with work experience. A doctor's role requires a huge commitment that can be fuelled by passion and determination.'

1 | Laughter is not always the best medicine
Studying medicine

This chapter mainly discusses studying medicine as an undergraduate course. For information on postgraduate courses, see the section entitled 'Postgraduate courses' on page 20.

Medical courses are carefully planned by the General Medical Council (GMC) to give students a wide range of academic and practical experience, which will lead to final qualification as a doctor. The main difference between medical schools is the method of teaching. At the end of the five-year course, students will – if they have met the high academic standards demanded – be awarded a Bachelor of Medicine or Bachelor of Medicine and Surgery (referred to as an MB or an MBBS, respectively). Many doctors come out with an MBChB – it all depends on which medical school you go to. As with dentistry, the ChB, i.e. Honours, is largely an honorary title. The MB is the Bachelor of Medicine while the ChB is the Bachelor of Surgery from the Latin *Baccalaureus Chirurgiae*.

It is well worth noting that, at this stage, doctors are graduates and have yet to do (if they so wish) a postgraduate doctoral degree such as a PhD. So they are, in the academic and philosophic sense, not doctors. However, when doctors specialise, it is then necessary to have a post-doctoral degree.

Teaching styles

The structure of all medical courses is similar, with most institutions offering two years of pre-clinical studies (often undertaken with dentistry students at the same university) followed by three years of clinical studies. However, schools differ in the ways in which they deliver the material, so it is very important to get hold of, and thoroughly read, the latest prospectuses of each university to which you are thinking of applying.

Medical courses can be classified as either traditional, problem-based learning (PBL) or integrated. Some places will even define six different types of medical course, adding case-based learning, enquiry-based learning and multi- or inter-professional-based learning. However, for the purposes of this book, we will take the standard approach and define the first three courses: traditional, problem-based and integrated learning.

The table below shows a list of the medical schools in the UK along with the teaching style they practise.

Table 2 Teaching styles

Medical school	Teaching style
University of Aberdeen	Integrated
University of Aston	Integrated
Barts and The London School of Medicine and Dentistry (Queen Mary University of London)	PBL
University of Birmingham	Integrated
Brighton and Sussex Medical School	Integrated
University of Bristol	Integrated
University of Buckingham	Integrated
University of Cambridge	Traditional
Cardiff University	PBL and CBL
University of Central Lancashire	Integrated
University of Dundee	Integrated
University of East Anglia	Integrated
University of Edinburgh	Integrated
University of Exeter	Integrated
University of Glasgow	Integrated
Hull York Medical School	PBL
Imperial College London	Integrated
Keele University	Integrated
King's College London	Integrated
University of Lancaster	PBL
University of Leeds	Integrated
University of Leicester	Integrated
University of Liverpool	Integrated
University of Manchester	PBL
Newcastle University	Integrated
University of Nottingham	Integrated
University of Oxford	Traditional
University of Plymouth	PBL
Queen's University Belfast	Traditional
Royal Free Hospital and University College London	Integrated
University of St Andrews	Integrated
St George's, University of London	Integrated
University of Sheffield	Integrated
University of Southampton	Integrated
Swansea University	Integrated
University of Warwick	Integrated

Traditional courses

This is the more long-established, lecture-based style, using didactic methods. The majority of these courses are subject-based ones, where lectures are the most appropriate way of delivering the information. It has to be said that these courses are a rarity today and are limited to establishments such as Cambridge, Oxford and Queen's University, Belfast, where there is a definite pre-clinical/clinical divide and the pre-clinical years are taught very rigidly in subjects.

TIP!

Find out more details about these traditional-based learning courses by going to the websites for the following medical schools:

- University of Oxford: www.medsci.ox.ac.uk
- University of Cambridge: www.medschl.cam.ac.uk

Course structure: Oxford (Traditional)

The six-year degree programme is designed to give students a comprehensive grounding in medical science, before applying it to a clinical environment. Teaching is delivered with an appreciation of academic research along the way.

First 5 terms

Students will all take the same compulsory courses. The principal focus will be on introducing fundamentals of the human body, and to the basic mechanisms underlying disease. There will then be a two-part examination:

Part I Examination

These core papers are: Organization of the Body, Physiology and Pharmacology, Biochemistry and Medical Genetics, Population Health 1 (Medical Sociology) and the Patient and Doctor course.

Part II Examination

Applied Physiology and Pharmacology, The Nervous System, Principles of Pathology, Psychology for Medicine and the Patient and Doctor course.

Last 4 terms

BA in Medical Sciences
In this section of the programme students currently choose from the

following advanced options: Neuroscience, Molecular Medicine, Cardiovascular, Renal & Respiratory Biology, Infection & Immunity and Cellular Physiology and Pharmacology. This will be in addition to a research project and extended essay, the focus of which will be a spirit of enquiry and critical thinking.

BA Examination
Principles of Clinical Anatomy

Clinical

In the final three years of the course, students will move into the clinical phase. There is a separate admissions process for this part of the course. The core curriculum will focus on preparing students for their Foundation Training, and in order to do this, there will be a wide range of subjects that will give students the opportunities to develop specialist knowledge, and explore research and presentational topics on subjects they may wish to focus on in their career. Years 4 and 5 will be subject to continuous, staged assessment.

Year 4: focus on honing of clinical skills

In this year, students will focus on the following: Patient and Doctor course II (+GP residential attachment), Laboratory Medicine, Rotations in Surgery and Medicine, Hospital attachment and Special study paper.

Year 5: focus on specialist clinical areas

In the following year, students will take part in six 8-week block rotations, in the following: Paediatrics, Psychiatry, Obstetrics & Gynaecology and Genito-urinary Medicine, Orthopaedics, A&E and Musculoskeletal Medicine, Clinical Geratology, Dermatology, Palliative Care, Public Health, Primary Care and Neurology and Neurosurgery, ENT, Ophthalmology.

Year 6: consolidation of skills and preparation for practice

In the final year, there will be an examination for BM BCh. This will take the form of senior rotations in medicine and surgery in Oxford and District General Hospitals, options in clinical specialities and Special study papers, a 10-week elective and work shadowing.

Source: www.medsci.ox.ac.uk/study/medicine/pre-clinical/structure
Reprinted with kind permission.

The above is an example as of 10 January 2018. Please note that the structure of the course may be subject to change at any time, and make sure to check the University's Medical Sciences Division website (www.medsci.ox.ac.uk) for the latest up-to-date information.

Problem-based learning (PBL)

The PBL course, commended by the GMC, was pioneered by medical schools such as Liverpool (which now offers an integrated course) and Manchester and subsequently taken up by a number of other medical schools such as Plymouth and Hull York. The course is taught with a patient-oriented approach. From year 1 onwards, students are heavily involved in clinical scenarios, with the focus on the student to demonstrate self-motivation and proactive, self-directed learning. This type of teaching/learning is designed to get away from the previous traditional 'spoon-fed' approach; therefore, those who are used to the spoon feeding of information may take some time to adjust.

Studying at Hull York Medical School

Hull York Medical School offers a different kind of undergraduate medicine programme, truly preparing students for real life as a junior doctor in the ever-changing NHS, through a combination of high quality, patient-centred teaching, clinician-led problem-based learning, and sustained clinical experience from week three of the programme.

As a partnership between the University of Hull and the University of York, the school is able to offer a unique breadth of sustained clinical experience, as well as access to the very best facilities, support networks, research opportunities and academic expertise that the two universities have to offer.

Training at Hull York Medical School is designed to develop the superior communication skills and confident, empathetic approach to delivering care that are the hallmark of the school's graduates. Problem-based learning and clinical skills training are facilitated by expert clinicians, so your studies are enhanced by the support and shared real-world experience of seasoned healthcare professionals. The school's commitment to small group teaching extends to clinical placements, where you will be taught first-hand in an intimate environment by very highly qualified clinicians, many of whom are practising consultants and senior specialists.

The dynamic, three-phase curriculum is founded on modern teaching methods, a solid grounding in the sciences and structured regular clinical contact, and is continually developed to reflect the latest educational methods and scientific research, as well as feedback from patients, NHS partners, students, alumni, tutors and faculty members.

The five-year course is divided into three phases:

- Phase I covers the first two years of the course and is based mainly on the Hull or York University campus;
- Phase II is largely based on a series of clinical placements throughout the region in a variety of healthcare settings;
- Phase III starts with your Elective, followed by further clinical placement experience and a final two-month assistantship working alongside junior doctors and a clinical team.

The tightly integrated curriculum is based on an understanding that disease doesn't exist in isolation, enabling you to make meaningful and practical connections between individual areas of study. You will explore topics through a range of themes and disciplines, each presented in a clinically relevant context, and supported through clinical experience, problem-based learning, lectures, clinical and communication skills classes, workshops and resource sessions. Returning to these topics throughout your training not only deepens your academic understanding, but also ensures that you are prepared on a practical level to respond appropriately and effectively in a clinical setting.

At the end of the five-year medical course, you will graduate with an MB BS degree, awarded jointly by the universities of Hull and York. This UK- and EU-recognised primary medical qualification combines two first degrees: Bachelor of Medicine and Bachelor of Surgery. In addition to the MB BS undergraduate programme, we offer postgraduate medical education, internationally recognised research degrees and a wide range of intercalation options. All of our students have the chance to study abroad during the elective period in Year 5 (Phase III), and the school has developed strong links with other medical schools outside the UK.

Source: www.hyms.ac.uk
Reprinted with kind permission of Hull York Medical School.
Please note that course details may be subject to change at any time, and make sure to check the university's website (www.hyms.ac.uk) for the most up-to-date information.

Integrated courses

Integrated courses are those where basic medical sciences are taught concurrently with clinical studies. Thus, this style is a compromise between a traditional course and a PBL course and, currently, is the most common type of medical course. Although these courses have patient contact from the start, there is huge variation in the amount of contact from school to school. In Year 1, contact is quite often limited to local community visits, with the amount of patient contact increasing as the years progress. In any case, most students are quite happy with having only limited contact with patients in the first year, as they feel that at this point they do not have a sufficient clinical knowledge base to approach patients on the wards.

Studying at Brighton and Sussex Medical School (integrated)

How is the course organised?

Phase 1: Years 1-2 (each divided into three, 10-week terms)

Your academic and clinical studies will be based primarily at both Brighton and Sussex University campuses at Falmer, using purpose-built teaching facilities including a modern anatomy laboratory, small and large group teaching spaces, clinical science laboratories and IT resource suites.

You will carry out two individual family studies: Year 1 with a family looking after a new baby; Years 2 and 3 by carrying out a longitudinal clerkship following a patient with dementia and their family.

The academic year is organised into three terms of 10 weeks each. About 25% of your learning at this stage will be clinically based and will include gaining experience in hospitals and primary and community medicine.

You will start to develop clinical skills in history taking, physical examination, diagnosis and effective communication with patients in a classroom setting and by spending time with a family looking after a new baby (Year 1), and carrying out a longitudinal clerkship following a patient with dementia (Years 2 and 3).

You will also study the normal and abnormal functioning of the human body using a system-based approach, with integrated modules covering the core biomedical and psychosocial sciences. Student-Selected Components (SSCs) will allow you to undertake individual studies and explore selected topics in depth, informed by the latest research.

Apart from core lectures and symposia, most Year 1 and 2 classes are taught in small groups. You will be supported by an academic tutor throughout Phase 1.

Phase 2: Years 3-4

Years 3 and 4 are based mainly in Brighton at the Royal Sussex County Hospital and Audrey Emerton Education Centre, and in

Haywards Heath at the Princess Royal Hospital. The Audrey Emerton provides comprehensive learning facilities, including a fully stocked medical library, computer suites, a clinical skills training area and teaching rooms for large and small group study. You will be supported by a clinical academic tutor throughout Years 3 to 5.

Year 3

It will start with a six-week course introducing clinical studies. At the heart of Year 3 are four eight-week, ward-based attachments in Medicine, Surgery, and Elderly Medicine and Psychiatry. You will consolidate your increasing clinical experience with your understanding of the underlying clinical, social science and public health issues through weekly teaching sessions on the scientific basis of medicine throughout Year 3, building on the core knowledge gained in Phase 1 and learning more about genetics, immunology, infectious diseases and therapeutics.

You will also gain further experience in safe prescribing of drugs, an essential skill for your medical career.

Student-Selected Components (SSCs) in Year 3 will deepen your understanding in an area of your choice from a variety of options in several short attachments in specialised areas, covering research, clinical effectiveness and medical humanities. You will maintain an ePortfolio that is similar to the one you will use as a junior doctor, which will help you to reflect on how your skills are developing.

Year 4

In Year 4, you will use all the skills developed over the preceding three years to work in more specialised clinical areas:

- General Practice
- Musculoskeletal Medicine and Surgery
- Ophthalmology and ENT
- Infectious Diseases, HIV GUM and Health Protection
- Dermatology
- Neurology and Neurosurgery
- Oncology, Haematology and Palliative Care
- Obstetrics and Gynaecology
- Paediatrics

The clinical focus in Year 4 is on understanding patients' integrated care and how primary, community and secondary care structures work together for the patient.

The other major component of Year 4 is an individual, year-long research project, supervised by a university or hospital research team, which can be laboratory based or more directly patient focused.

Online

In Years 4 and 5 your learning will be supported by the online learning tool CAPSULE, a custom-built website and app. CAPSULE provides you with 670 clinical case studies and more than 3,500 questions mapped to the medical curriculum. After completing a case, you will be provided with instant feedback, to maximise your learning.

Phase 3: Year 5

Year 5 starts with a 24-week series of placements that will provide intense clinical and professional preparation for your foundation years. Throughout the year, you will develop your clinical skills through direct patient contact and by using clinical skills laboratories and simulators.

As a student assistant, you will undertake clinical attachments in different regional locations including Chichester, Eastbourne, Hastings, Haywards Heath, Redhill, Worthing. Your learning will be based on a close involvement with routine clinical cases, acting as a member of the clinical team in medicine, emergency medicine, elderly medicine, surgery, general practice and psychiatry. Central to your study will be the assessment, diagnosis and treatment of patients presenting to these different areas of practice.

You will take part in a seminar programme and a range of mini conferences, which cover topics such as NHS structure, patient safety, leadership skills and advanced communication and ethical skills.

Following your final examinations, you will undertake a four-week clinical elective period to experience healthcare in another environment in the UK or abroad. You will then undergo a Preparation for Practice module that will build on all you have done in the previous years so you are well prepared for life as a foundation doctor. At the start of Year 5 you will also apply for your foundation year training posts, and later in the year take the national Situational Judgement Test and Prescribing Safety Assessment.

Foundation Year training

Your degree in medicine will equip you with the knowledge and clinical and personal skills you will need to progress to the next stages of your training. Wherever you undertake foundation training, you will have close educational supervision and continue with your ePortfolio.

> **The intercalated degree**
>
> Subject to performance, you may be offered the opportunity to undertake an intercalated degree between Years 3 and 4, allowing you to study an area of interest in greater depth. Intercalation means taking a year out of your normal medical curriculum to study for an extra degree, which may be a BSc or a Masters degree. This will lengthen your studies by a year but provide you with rigorous training in research methods, and may allow you to publish your findings and attend scientific meetings and conferences.
>
> The extra degree, research and publication will all add to your CV and make you more competitive for your next career step.
>
> Source: www.bsms.ac.uk/undergraduate/our-course/course-structure.aspx
> Reprinted with the kind permission of Brighton and Sussex Medical School.

Case-based learning

This is not the same as problem-based learning, though its ideals are the same. Unlike PBL, which is focused on problem-based scenarios, case-based learning looks at case studies within a clinical environment. It is actually quite a common route for a lot of international medical schools, though Cardiff University is an example of a UK medical school that uses it, similarly the University of Glasgow and University of Liverpool makes use of it to some extent. It is a popular way of learning, with a US poll among 286 students and 31 faculties displaying an 89% preference for the CBL teaching methods.

The style of teaching will be in small groups and utilises clinical cases to elicit interest and discussion in a specific part of the course curriculum. Within these sessions, activities will be carried out with a plenary session at the end for students to share their experiences and discuss the application of them in the future.

It is expected this type of learning will become more popular in the UK sooner rather than later with more universities starting to use this style of teaching.

Intercalated degrees

Students who perform well in the examinations at the end of their preclinical studies (year 2 or 3) often take up the opportunity to complete an intercalated degree. An intercalated degree gives you the opportunity to incorporate a further degree (BSc or BA) into your medical course. This is normally a one-year project, during which students have the opportunity to investigate a chosen topic in much more depth, producing a final written thesis before rejoining the main course. Usually, a range of degrees are available to choose from, such as those from the traditional sciences, i.e. biochemistry, anatomy, physiology, or in topics as different as medical law, ethics, journalism and/or history of medicine.

Further features of an intercalated degree include the following.

- Anatomy continues to be taught using whole-body dissection.
- Students will complete two degrees over the five years: the Bachelor of Medical Sciences in year 3 and the medical degrees (Bachelor of Medicine, Bachelor of Surgery) in year 5.
- The research component of the BMedSci degree provides students with excellent experience in research, with the opportunity of publishing papers.
- A professional approach is taken to training in that it uses procedures that are employed in the assessment of doctors after they graduate.
- The clinical training component of the course sees the amalgamation of students from the year 4 and 5 courses, which enhances the educational experience for both groups.

Why intercalate?

- It gives you the chance to study a particular subject in depth.
- It gives you the chance to be involved in research or lab work, particularly if you are interested in research later on.
- It gives you an advantage over other candidates if you later decide to specialise; for example, intercalating in anatomy would be useful if you wish to pursue a career in surgery.

Why not intercalate?

- The main drawback is the extra cost and time involved in taking a detour in your studies. This needs to be considered carefully.
- You could forget some of the things you've learned in the previous years of your medical degree, and thus will need to spend time reacquainting yourself with the forgotten material.

The following is an example of King's College London's (KCL) intercalated degree offering. It is a one-year BSc programme giving students an option to study related subjects in more detail. This programme is taken after the second, third or fourth year of study and is flag-posted to anyone who is looking to work in medical research after they have completed their course.

Example of an intercalated degree

King's College London offers one of the broader programmes at university, including:

- Anatomy, Developmental and Human Biology
- Craniofacial and Stem Cell Biology
- Endocrinology: Clinical and Molecular
- Forensic Psychiatry, Criminal Behaviour and Law
- Gerontology
- Global Health
- History of Medicine
- Human Nutrition and Metabolism
- Imaging Sciences
- Infectious Diseases and Immunobiology
- Medical Genetics
- Neuroscience
- Pharmacology
- Philosophy
- Physiology
- Psychology
- Regenerative Medicine & Innovation Technology
- Women's Health.

The list is an example as of December 2017. Please note that the intercalated courses available are subject to change at any time, and ensure to check the university website (www.kcl.ac.uk) for the most up-to-date information.

Source: www.kcl.ac.uk/study/subject-areas/intercalated/
intercalated-bsc-courses.aspx
Reprinted with kind permission from King's College London

TIP!

Websites with further information about intercalated degrees:

- www.intercalate.co.uk
- www.smd.qmul.ac.uk/undergraduate/intercalated (Barts and The London School of Medicine and Dentistry)
- www.kcl.ac.uk/study/subject-areas/intercalated/intercalated-bsc-courses.aspx

Taking an elective

Towards the end of the course there is often the opportunity to take an elective study period, usually for two months, when students are expected to undertake a short project but are free to travel to any hospital or clinic in the world that is approved by their university. This gives you the opportunity to practise medicine anywhere in the world during your clinical years. For example, electives range from running clinics in developing countries to accompanying flying doctors in Australia. Students see this as an opportunity to do some travelling and visit exotic locations far from home before they qualify. You can also, if you want, opt to do an elective at home. If you want to know more about this, go to www.worktheworld.co.uk.

Postgraduate courses

There is a huge variety of opportunities and courses for further post-graduate education and training in medicine. This reflects the array of possible areas for specialisation. Medical schools and hospitals run a wide range of postgraduate programmes, which include further clinical and non-clinical training and research degree programmes.

Advice and guidance are available from the Royal College of Physicians (RCP) (www.rcplondon.ac.uk) and the individual universities. As before, you will need to check the prospectuses of individual universities for the most up-to-date information.

Examples of postgraduate courses

The following postgraduate courses are offered by the University of Nottingham:

- Applied Sport and Exercise Medicine (MSc)
- Assisted Reproduction Technology (MMedSci)
- Cancer Immunology and Biotechnology (MSc)
- Clinical Academic Training Programme (CATP)
- Forensic and Criminological Psychology (MSc by research)
- Forensic psychology (DForenPsy)
- Health psychology (MSc/PhD)
- Management Psychology (MSc)
- Medical Education (MMedSci)
- Mental Health Research (MSc)
- Microbiology and Immunology (MSc)
- Molecular Pathology (MSc by research)
- Musculoskeletal Sport Science and Health (MSc/PGDip)

- Occupational Psychology (MSc)
- Oncology (MSc)
- Public Health (International Health) (MPH)
- Rehabilitation Psychology (MSc)
- Sports and Exercise Medicine (MSc)
- Stem Cell Technology (MSc)
- Work and Organisational Psychology (MSc)
- Workplace Health and Wellbeing (Distance E-Learning MSc).

Source: www.nottingham.ac.uk
Reprinted with kind permission of The University of Nottingham

As you will see from the example course descriptions, all medical school courses cover the same essential information but can vary widely in their teaching styles; this is an important point to consider when choosing which course to apply to. Chapter 2 has further guidance on what to consider when choosing your university and course.

Case study

Emily joined medical school at the University of East Anglia. While studying for a philosophy degree, she realised that medicine was what she wanted to dedicate her time to and therefore went back to college to study A levels in one year.

'My route to medicine has been non-standard. There was something about a philosophy degree that gave me clarity of thought, ironically. I wasn't sure exactly what to undertake as a career when I left school, though learning about medical philosophy made me think, perhaps my career was in this particular sector.

'So I went back to college in order to study the required subjects for the degree. This was not the hard bit for me, it was the UKCAT that I found difficult. You get so used to thinking in one way that this exam completely reanalysed how I should approach topics. The best tip to give anyone: you cannot practise enough. This is a true examination of your brain and ability to think under pressure, therefore prepare as soon as you can if you want to do well in it. Speaking to other people, I discovered they all got scored highly on their test – much higher than me – and I did not do badly, so that shows how competitive it is.

'I joined medicine late so I thought my priorities would be different to those of the younger students; however, I have been amazed by how focused everyone is, which is testament to how demanding this course is. I do find it inspiring how supportive everyone is towards a common goal. The work is tough and the hours should not be underestimated, although the reward is worth it. The satisfaction I get from the knowledge and understanding is inspiring. The course is not overwhelming though and, strange as it may seem, I almost expected more work.

'The first term was intensive, though that may just have been because it was the start of a new course. Work and placements quickly settle into routine. I am on an Integrated course so I am grateful of the PBL elements to balance the theory. I really value the practical application at this early stage of the course because there is no substitute to working with the patients and seeing how unglamorous medicine is.

'My advice to any student: be forensic with your work experience, use it as a chance to fully understand the profession you are aiming to be part of once graduated; practise for interviews, because interviews are artificial scenarios and the more help you can get is worth it; and don't panic – that is one of the principal conditions of being a doctor – listen to what you are being told and respond calmly, even when under pressure.'

2 | Doctor, doctor ...
Applying to study medicine

Getting an interview is essential because most medical schools issue conditional offers only after their admissions panel has met you. The evidence that the selector uses when he or she makes the choice to call you for interview or reject you is your UCAS application, which means that your application is the first vital step in getting into medical school. This chapter will guide you through the different parts of your application, including choosing where to apply, admissions tests and academic ability.

Some sections of the application are purely factual (your name, address, exam results, etc.). There is also a section where you enter your choice of medical schools. The personal statement section gives you an opportunity to write about yourself, and there is a space for your teacher to write a reference describing your strengths and weaknesses. Later in this book, you will find advice on how to fill in these sections and how to influence your referee, but first let's consider what happens, or might happen, to your application.

What happens to your application

Typically, a medical school might receive between 1,500 and 2,000 applications, almost all of which will arrive in September and October. The applications are distributed to the selectors, who have to decide which applicants to recommend for interview. The selectors will usually be busy doctors, and the task of selecting promising candidates means a good deal of extra work for them, on top of the usual demands of their full-time jobs. Most of the candidates will have been predicted grades that will allow them to be considered but the medical school can interview perhaps only 15% to 25% of them.

A high proportion of applicants will have good GCSE results and predicted grades at A level of AAA or higher. (NB: nearly all universities now ask for three A grades and some for at least one A* grade.) They will also have undertaken some voluntary work or work-shadowing. In order to decide who should be called for interview, the selectors will have to make a decision based solely on the information provided by you and your school. If you are not called for interview, you will not be offered a place at that medical school (apart from in the case of the

University of Edinburgh, which tends not to base its decisions on face-to-face interviews). If your application does not convince the selector that you are the right sort of person to be a doctor, he or she will reject you. However outstanding your personal qualities are, unless your application is convincing, you will not be called for interview. This part of the guide is designed to maximise your chances of getting the interview even under the worst circumstances.

Deciding where to apply

There are currently 34 medical schools or university departments of medicine in the UK that are recognised by the Medical Schools Council (MSC). However, please note that Durham's school of Medicine, Pharmacy and Health relocated to Newcastle University, so from 2017 prospective medical students are no longer able to apply to Durham. We do not discuss the London School of Hygiene and Tropical Medicine. The University of Buckingham is counted as number 35, though it is a private university, University of Aston as of 2017 and there is also the University of Central Lancashire (UCLan), which is purely for international students; neither of these appear on the MSC list. However, Swansea University and Warwick Medical School now appear on the MSC list although they offer Graduate Entry programmes (A101) only. The universities on the list offer a range of options for students wishing to study medicine:

- five- or six-year MBBS or MBChB courses (UCAS codes A100 or A106)
- four-year accelerated graduate-entry courses (A101, A102 or A109)
- six-year courses that include a 'pre-med' year (A103 or A104).

Entry requirements of all medical schools are summarised in Table 12 (see pages 206–208).

You can apply to up to four medical schools in one application cycle. In deciding which ones to eliminate, you may find the following points helpful.

- **Grades and retakes.** If you are worried that you will not achieve AAA grades (minimum) the first time round, include at least three schools that accept retake candidates (see Table 13 on pages 209–210). The reason for this is that if you make a good impression at interview this year, you may not need to face a second interview at your next attempt. You will also be able to show loyalty by applying twice to the same school. Many medical schools will consider second-time applicants only if they applied to them originally.
- **Interviews.** Almost all medical schools interview A level candidates; some use traditional panel interviews, while others use Multiple Mini Interviews (MMIs). Each school's interview policy is shown in Table 13 (see pages 209–210).

- **Location and socialising.** You may be attracted to the idea of being at a campus university rather than at one of the medical schools that are not located on the campuses of their affiliated universities. One reason for this may be that you would like to mix with students from a wide variety of disciplines and that you will enjoy the intellectual and social cross-fertilisation. The trouble with this theory is that medical students work longer hours than most other students and tend to form a clique. Be warned: in reality you could find that you have little time to mix with non-medics.
- **Course structure.** While all the medical schools are well equipped and provide a high standard of teaching, there are real differences in the way the courses are taught and examined and you will not find two the same. Specifically, the majority offer an integrated course in which students see patients at an early stage and certainly before the formal clinical part of the course. The other main distinction is between systems-based courses (e.g. Manchester and Liverpool), which teach medicine in terms of the body's systems (e.g. the cardiovascular system), and subject-based courses (e.g. Oxford and Cambridge), which teach in terms of the fundamental subjects (anatomy, biochemistry, etc.).
- **Teaching style.** The style of teaching can also vary from place to place. See pages 8–17 for more information on PBL, integrated and traditional approaches to teaching.
- **Intercalated degrees and electives.** Another difference in the courses offered concerns the opportunities for an intercalated Honours BSc and electives. The intercalated BSc scheme allows students to tack on one further year of study either to the end of the two-year pre-clinical course or as an integrated part of a six-year course. Successful completion of this year, which may be used to study a wide variety of subjects, confers a BSc degree qualification. Electives are periods of work experience away from the medical school and, in some cases, abroad. See pages 17–22 for more information.

When choosing where to apply you should consult the medical schools' websites and prospectuses. Once you have narrowed the choice down to about 10 or 12, it is worth writing to these for a copy of their prospectus (these will be sent to you free of charge) or taking a good look at their websites, from which you can download a copy of the prospectus.

The fifth choice

Although you can apply to a total of five institutions through UCAS, you may apply to only four medical schools; if you enter more than four, your application will be rejected. The question is: what should you do with the other slot? The medical schools will assure you that you can apply for other, non-medical courses without jeopardising your application to medicine, but we would advise you to think carefully before doing so, for the reasons given below.

- There's no point in thinking about alternatives if you really want to become a doctor.
- If you are unlucky and receive no conditional offers for medicine, you may have to accept an offer from your 'insurance' course.
- You might find it harder to convince your interviewers that you are completely committed to a career in medicine if you appear to be happy to accept a place to study, say, chemical engineering or archaeology. The selectors cannot see what your other choices are but you will find it difficult to write a personal statement that appeals to both medical admissions tutors and those for another subject and you risk being rejected by all of your choices if you try to cover all subjects in your personal statement.

The one reason to put a non-medical choice on your form is if you are not prepared to wait a year if your application is unsuccessful, and you intend to enter medicine as a graduate (see page 163).

Are there any other options?

Yes, and a very good one. It is often difficult to commit to a three-year degree course in something else when all you ever wanted to do is study medicine. Therefore many students apply for biomedical courses as their fifth choice. If they are unsuccessful in their initial application this has often proved a way into medical school in future years.

A biomedical sciences course that may be a suitable fifth choice for medicine is the two-year BSc run by Medipathways College in London. This BSc is designed specially for those who wish to study medicine or dentistry (as opposed to becoming a scientist).

- This two-year course is very medically focused (e.g. teaching through clinical scenarios), so it will not feel like you are studying something completely different to medicine for two years.
- Preparation for medical school (UKCAT, interviews, etc.) is offered.
- The BSc is accepted by virtually all UK medical schools for their four- or five-year courses. In 2015–2017, 60% of their graduates secured a place in the UK (national average is approximately 10%). Of those obtaining a First class degree, 100% have secured a medical school placement in the UK.
- Those with predicted grades of AAA can join a one-year pre-medical course and then progress onto the two-year BSc if they do not secure a place in medicine after first year.
- You will have access to unique resources, such as student membership at the Royal Society of Medicine.
- In the event that you are unsuccessful with your application after graduating, there is an option to study on a four-year course abroad.

For further information, please visit: www.medipathways.com.

To BSc ... or not to BSc?

Here we discuss courses such as biomedicine, biochemistry and other science degrees related to medicine. Many students reach this cross-road initially during the application process when considering their fifth option or if they don't get the offers they expected and intend to apply for medicine as a graduate two or three years later.

To BSc or not to BSc is a very tricky question to answer as ultimately no one else can answer it for you. Here are a few pros and cons for you to consider that might help make up your mind:

Cons

● You might spend a whole three years on a course you never really wanted to study.
● Three years of study will add additional cost and time before actually getting into medical school.
● Entry to medical school after graduating is not guaranteed.
● If admitted to undergraduate medical school only, you will still have to study for five more years.
● You might lose focus on medicine if you study something else first.
● You may not get the student funding and help towards fees, compared with if you go straight after A levels.

Pros

● Many BSc degrees are in biomedical or medical school – if you don't enjoy this, then are you sure you would enjoy medicine, which is not that different? There are also two-year BSc courses designed for medicine.
● Medicine is a life-long commitment, so two to three years of additional study should not worry you. Becoming a good doctor is a journey, not a target.
● Although entry to medical school is not guaranteed, some BSc courses do offer a very secure pathway to overseas medical schools in the event you don't get into the UK.
● Applying as a graduate certainly makes your medical school application stronger as you have matured as an individual and academically.
● Having a BSc as well as a medical degree may enhance your chances to get the medical job you desire – a reason why many medical students intercalate.

Applying to Oxbridge medical schools

Oxbridge is in a separate category because, if getting into most medical schools is difficult, entry into Oxford or Cambridge is even more so (the extra hurdles facing students wishing to apply to Oxford or Cambridge are discussed in *Getting into Oxford & Cambridge*, another guide in this series). The general advice given here also applies to Oxbridge, but the competition is intense, and before you include either university on your UCAS application you need to be confident that you can achieve the entrance standard grades (A*A*A at Cambridge and A*AA at Oxford) at A level and that you will interview well.

> **TIP!**
>
> You should discuss an application to Oxford or Cambridge with your teachers at an early stage.

You cannot apply to both Oxford and Cambridge in your application and your teachers will advise you whether to apply to either. You would need a good reason to apply to Oxbridge against the advice of your teachers and it certainly is not worth applying on the 'off chance' of getting in. By doing so you will simply waste one of your valuable four choices.

> **What the selector looks for**
>
> Most medical schools use a form that the selector fills in as he or she reads through your application. Have a look at the example form given in Figure 1; the next part of the chapter will examine each heading on this form in more detail.

Academic ability

GCSE results: points total and breadth of subjects

By the time you read this you will probably have chosen your GCSE subjects or even taken them. If not, here are some points to consider.

- Medical school selectors like to see breadth. Try to take as many GCSE subjects as possible. Try to take at least eight, but if your school places restrictions on the choice or number of GCSEs you take, make this clear in your personal statement.
- You will almost certainly need to study two science/maths subjects at A level, and you will need to study chemistry. There is a big gap between GCSE and A level. If you have the choice, don't make that jump even harder by studying combined or integrated science rather than the single science subjects. If your school will not allow you to study the single subjects, you should consider taking extra lessons during the summer holiday after your GCSE exams.
- Medical school selectors look at applicants' GCSE grades in considerable detail, arguably more so now in England where the A level has been decoupled so that the AS is a standalone qualification.

This means that in most cases, universities can no longer use the AS examination indicator as representative of how students will fare at A level. Many medical schools ask for a 'good' set of GCSE results. What does this mean? Well, it varies from university to university, but under the old-style grading system a minimum of five A/B grades at GCSE plus good grades in English language and maths are likely to be required. Some medical schools ask for a minimum of six A or A* grades at GCSE.

MEDICAL INTERVIEW SELECTION FORM

Name: UCAS number:
Age at entry: Gap year?:
Selector: Date:

SELECTION CRITERIA COMMENTS

1 Academic (score out of 10)
GCSE results/AS grades/A level predictions
UKCAT/BMAT result

2 Commitment (score out of 10)
Genuine interest in medicine?
Relevant work experience?
Community involvement?

3 Personal (score out of 10)
Range of interests?
Involvement in school activities?
Achievements and/or leadership?
Referee supports application?

Total score (maximum of 30):

Recommendation of selector: Interview   Score 25–30
                                 Reserve list   Score 16–24
                                 Rejection   Score 0–15

Further comments (if any):

Figure 1 Sample candidate selection form

GCSE reforms

In the same way as their A level counterparts, GCSEs are being reformed in phases. In September 2015, new GCSEs were formed in English language, English literature and mathematics, with the first examinations in May 2017. The phasing in of the new GCSEs has been over two years with the majority of 9–1 GCSEs and IGCSEs available for examination in May 2018; more information of what will be available for examination in which year up until June 2019 is available on www.gov.uk/government/publications/get-the-facts-gcse-and-a-level-reform/get-the-facts-gcse-reform.

Under the GCSE reforms, the new GCSEs use numbers instead of grades, and you will be expected to achieve 8s and 9s in your examinations. NB GCSE reforms are now extending to IGCSEs in core subjects, such as mathematics and science, with the first examinations in June 2018. The reforms discussed in this book mostly concern the system in England; the rest of the UK is undergoing reforms of their own, information on which can be found on the UCAS website: www.ucas.com/advisers/guides-and-resources/qualification-reform.

In addition to the grades required at A level, all of the universities specify the minimum grades that they require at GCSE. This varies from university to university, but it is unlikely that you will be considered unless you have at least five or six GCSEs, including science, English and maths, taken at one sitting and at grade A/B or 7/8 and above (check specific university websites for the exact requirements). If you have already taken your GCSEs and achieved disappointing grades, you must resign yourself to working exceptionally hard from the first day of your A level course. You will also need to convince your referee that the GCSE grades are not an indicator of low grades at A level, so that this can be mentioned in your reference.

If your grades fall below these requirements you need to get your referee to comment on them, to explain either why you underperformed (illness, family disruption, etc.) or why they expect your A level performance to be better than your GCSE grades indicate.

A level reform

In a previous post as Education Secretary, Michael Gove announced his intention to make significant changes to the A level system. These educational reforms came into effect in September 2015 and are ongoing. The aim behind the reforms was to move towards a linear model, thereby creating students who are better equipped for university as a result of a rigorous final examination as the culmination of two years' study. Students sit examinations at the end of the first year but these do not count for the final result, as A levels have been decoupled and the AS is now a standalone qualification.

The reforms are different in each country of the UK: www.ucas.com/advisers/guides-and-resources/qualification-reform. The changes discussed here apply to A levels for students sitting the qualifications set by English examination boards, but there are separate educational reforms taking place in Wales and Northern Ireland (as listed on the UCAS website).

The reforms were implemented in three phases.

Phase One: Art and Design, Biology, Business Studies, Chemistry, Economics, English Literature, History, Physics, Psychology and Sociology. These subjects were available for first teaching in September 2015.

Phase Two: Dance, Drama and Theatre, Geography, Music, Modern Foreign Languages (French, German, Spanish), Physical Education and Religious Studies. These subjects were available for first teaching from September 2016.

Phase Three: Accounting, Archaeology, Classical Civilisation, Design and Technology – Product Design, Design and Technology – Fashion Design and Development, Environmental Science, Further Maths, Government and Politics, History of Art, Information and Communications Technology, Law, Maths, Media Studies, Philosophy and Statistics. These subjects were available for first teaching in September 2017.

More information on what will be available for examination in which year until 2019 can be found at www.gov.uk/government/publications/get-the-facts-gcse-and-a-level-reform/get-the-facts-as-and-a-level-reform.

The AS and A2 (now an historic term) qualifications have been decoupled, which means that the new AS no longer counts towards the A level. Not every school is offering the decoupled AS under the new system. Some schools are offering the option to study a subject at AS as a qualification in its own right alongside the first year of A levels, while other schools are only offering A levels over two years. Most universities have said that they will not be using AS grades in offers anymore and stated that students will not be at a disadvantage if it is not possible to take an AS at their school or college, provided they meet the A level requirements; however, you should check university websites for their individual requirements.

What impact does this have on you? Well, it depends on the positioning of the school. The school has a choice whether to enter students for exams at the end of the first year. If it does this, it runs the risk of raising your profile before you are ready, as universities may regard your results as an indicator of your progress. That said, the new AS, though it will not count for the final examination results, would be good practice.

Therefore, in both eventualities, even though the new A level is a two-year qualification, you must make sure you treat any exams you take in your first year as formal qualifications. As said previously, GCSE grades are more important than ever before and, obvious as it sounds, you need to manage the transition from GCSE to the first year of sixth form more effectively than in recent years, as there is no room for slow starts.

AS exams: do they matter?

Under the outgoing AS and A2 level system, there was a lot of pressure on you from the start of your two-year courses, since not only did the AS grades appear on your application, but also many of the medical schools would specify minimum grade requirements. Even those that did not would consciously or subconsciously use them as an indicator of a candidate's likely A level grades. The other thing that had to be borne in mind was that a low score at AS – C grades, say – was unlikely to lead to AAA at A level since an AS contributed up to 50% of the total A level marks, and so selectors may have doubted that the predicted grades (see below) were achievable.

With the new system, the term 'AS' still exists, though under the reforms it no longer counts towards the full A level. Remember that how well you do is important from the start. Even though universities no longer have an explicit AS grade requirement, Lancaster, for example, will judge a candidate's offer on whether they have been able to sit a fourth AS exam at their school or not (see Table 12, pages 206–208), and in reality they are a useful indicator as to how the overall A level will go. Equally, if you sit AS exams, those marks, while they will not count in a full A level qualification, may well be used by universities as an indicator of your likely A level grades. The advice is, make sure you are taking the subject because it is your choice to do that and not because you feel you should or have to take another subject.

A level predictions

Your choice of A levels

You will see from Table 12 (pages 206–208) that most medical schools now ask for just two science/maths subjects at A level. They all require chemistry and/or biology so you need to choose either physics or maths if you wish to apply to a medical school that requires three science/maths subjects. There are three important considerations.

1. Choose subjects that you are good at. You must be capable of an A grade as a minimum requirement. If you aren't sure, ask your teachers.
2. Choose subjects that will help you in your medical course; life at medical school is tough enough as it is without having to learn new subjects from scratch.

3. While it is acceptable to choose a non-scientific third subject that you enjoy and that will provide you with an interesting topic of conversation at your interview, you should be careful not to choose subjects such as art, which is practical rather than academic, though as a fourth subject it is viable. General studies is not acceptable either. However, students who can cope with the differing demands of arts and sciences at A level have an advantage in that they can demonstrate breadth.

So what combination of subjects should you choose? In addition to chemistry/biology and another science at A level, you might also consider subjects such as psychology, sociology or a language. In the reforms, psychology as a subject became more mathematical, as well as scientific; as such, the University of Sheffield will now regard it as a second science subject in their grade offers. The point to bear in mind when you are making your choices is that you need high grades, so do not pick a subject that sounds interesting, such as Italian, if you are not good at languages. Similarly, although an A level in further mathematics might look good on your UCAS application, you will need to consider if it is actually something universities want you to have. You will need to check the individual requirements; most medical schools will indicate preferred A level subjects in addition to science A levels.

Taking four A levels

There's no harm in doing more than three A levels (and an AS exam, if offered by your school), but there is really no advantage to it; and do drop any additional qualifications if there is a danger of them pulling down your overall grades. Medical schools will not include the fourth A level in any conditional offers they make.

If you are taking the International Baccalaureate, then you should still be aiming to take biology and chemistry as these are the subjects required for undergraduate study. However, some universities specify chemistry and one of maths, biology, human biology and physics. If you are not taking these subjects you should be considering what makes you think you will be able to cope on a medicine course. For Scottish students, you are expected to have at least two Advanced Highers and three Highers, with biology and chemistry and usually either mathematics or physics as well to at least Higher level; Imperial College, for example, asks for five Highers and three Advanced Highers to A grade standard. Overall, students should be aiming for majority A grades in Highers and Advanced Highers, though AB at Advanced Highers is accepted, or even BB in the case of the University of Edinburgh, for example.

The prediction

The selector will look for a grade prediction in the reference that your teacher writes about you. Your teacher will make a prediction based on the reports of your subject teachers, your GCSE grades and, most importantly, the results of any exams taken at the end of year 12.

Consequently, it is vital that you work hard during the first year of A levels. Only by doing so will you get the reference you need. If there is any reason or excuse to explain why you did badly at GCSE or did not work hard in year 12, you must make sure that the teacher writing your reference knows about it and includes it in the reference. The most common reasons for poor performance are illness and problems at home (e.g. illness of a close relation or family breakdown).

The bottom line is that you need to persuade your school that you are on track for grades of AAA or higher, depending on where you are applying. Convincing everyone else usually involves convincing yourself!

Aptitude tests

Some universities ask applicants to sit aptitude tests as part of the application process. These tests include the UKCAT and BMAT tests.

UKCAT (the UK Clinical Aptitude Test)

The UKCAT has been adopted by 26 universities as part of their admissions procedures, and helps them make an informed choice between the highest candidates for undergraduate medical study. It is designed to ensure that students have the mental capabilities, attitude and professional conduct required for a career in the medical field. It is not a test of your curriculum knowledge or any scientific background. The UKCAT tests thought processes and as such cannot be revised for. It is a computer-based test but needs to be sat at an official centre.

Test centres can be found in many locations worldwide. Registration is open between May and September and you can sit the test between early July and early October, though the earlier you take it, the better. If there is a problem with your attending any of these centres, you should consult the UKCAT website (www.ukcat.ac.uk). If you have any disabilities or additional needs that require you to have extra time in examinations, it is important that you register for the UKCATSEN instead of the regular test. If you require special access arrangements for examinations, then you should directly contact Pearson VUE customer services to discuss these arrangements before you book the test.

There are five sections to the UKCAT. These sections are based on a set of skills that medical (and dental) schools believe are vital to be successful as a medical practitioner. The five sections are listed below.

1. **Verbal Reasoning.** Candidates are provided with a piece of text that they have to analyse and answer questions on.
2. **Decision Making.** This test assesses a candidate's ability to apply logic to reach a decision or conclusion, evaluate arguments and analyse statistical information.
3. **Quantitative Reasoning.** The candidate's ability to deal with numerical questions is tested.
4. **Abstract Reasoning.** Candidates have to draw relationships from written information.
5. **Situational Judgement.** This tests candidates' ability to comprehend real-world situations and to identify critical factors and appropriate behaviour in handling them.

The test lasts two hours. Those candidates with special educational needs take the UKCATSEN and are given longer (about 25% more time) for each set of questions.

Table 3 Timings for UKCAT/UKCATSEN

Section	Items	Standard Test Time	Extra Time/UKCATSEN
Verbal Reasoning	44 items	22 minutes	27.5 minutes
Decision Making	29 items	32 minutes	40 minutes
Quantitative Reasoning	36 items	25 minutes	31.25 minutes
Abstract Reasoning	55 items	14 minutes	17.25 minutes
Situational Judgement	690 items	27 minutes	33.75 minutes
Total time		120 minutes	150 minutes

Dates

A list of important dates regarding the UKCAT exam can be found at www.ukcat.ac.uk. For those students wishing to apply for entry in 2019, the most important ones are as follows:

- registration opens: 2 May 2018
- testing begins: 3 July 2018
- registration deadline: 5pm on 19 September 2018
- last testing date: 3 October 2018

Universities that require the UKCAT

Table 4 on the following page shows the UK universities that require students to sit the UKCAT as part of their application process.

Table 4 Medical schools requiring UKCAT admissions test

Medical school	UCAS course code
University of Aberdeen	A100
University of Aston	A100
Barts and The London School of Medicine and Dentistry	A100, A101, A110
University of Birmingham	A100
University of Bristol	A100, A108
University of Cardiff	A100, A104
University of Dundee	A100, A104
University of East Anglia	A100, A104
University of Edinburgh	A100
University of Exeter	A100
University of Glasgow	A100
Hull York Medical School	A100
Keele University (for domestic applicants)	A100, A104
King's College London	A100, A101, A102
University of Leicester	A100
University of Liverpool	A100
University of Manchester	A104, A106
Newcastle University	A100, A101
University of Nottingham	A100, A108
University of Plymouth (Peninsula Schools of Medicine and Dentistry)	A100
Queen's University Belfast	A100
University of Sheffield	A100, A104
University of Southampton	A100, A101, A102
University of St Andrews	A100
St George's, University of London	A100, A900
University of Warwick Graduate Entry	A101

Preparation

Although the UKCAT website tries to discourage students from doing any preparation for the test other than sitting the practice tests available online, students who have sat the test in the past have found that the more practice they had on timed IQ-type tests, the better prepared they felt. In this chapter you will find practice questions for each section.

General hints

- Use the practice tests provided on the following pages to familiarise yourself with the type of questions that are asked and the time constraints in the test.
- Most candidates do not complete all sections in the test so don't worry if you don't. Use the practice test to ensure that you know

how to pace yourself. Try to answer all of the questions but don't worry if you don't get to the end of each section.

- There is a point for each right answer, but no points are deducted for wrong answers.
- Try not to leave blanks. If you really can't work out the answer, it is better to eliminate the answers that you know to be wrong and then make your best guess from those that are left.
- Leave enough time to guess the remaining questions. Our advice would be one minute.
- Be aware that you must read the whole screen of the question that you are on, otherwise you cannot move on to the next question or go back to any of the questions you have answered. There are both vertical and horizontal scroll bars.
- Finally, it is most important that you stay calm in the test. Prepare yourself, pace yourself and move on if you're struggling with particular questions. It is inevitable that you will find some questions and some sections easier than others.

Below follows a summary of each subtest, with sample questions provided courtesy of Kaplan Test Prep.

Verbal Reasoning

The Verbal Reasoning test is designed to assess your ability to read and think carefully about information, using comprehension passages to get you to draw specific conclusions from the information presented. The test is based upon the verbal reasoning skills required of doctors to take on board often complex information, to analyse it and then to communicate in simple terms to patients and their families. There are 11 text passages which all have four questions to answer. Some questions will test your comprehension skills by asking you to answer 'true', 'false' or 'can't tell'. The other type of question tests your critical response and will look for you to draw a conclusion. You will be presented with an incomplete statement or a question and four response options. You need to pick the most suitable response.

UKCAT Verbal Reasoning Practice Questions

Subtest length: 44 questions (11 sets of 4 questions)
Subtest timing: 21 minutes (2 minutes per set)
Sample length: 4 questions
Sample timing: 2 minutes

In September 1997, Scotland held a referendum on the question of devolution. Over 60 per cent of eligible voters went to the polls, and they voted in favour of both questions on the ballot-paper. On the first question, asking whether there should be a

---

Scottish Parliament, 74.3 per cent of voters agreed, including a majority in favour in every Scottish local authority area. On the second question, asking whether that Parliament should have tax-varying powers, 63.5 per cent of voters agreed, including a majority in favour in every Scottish local authority area except Orkney and Dumfries & Galloway. In response to the results of this referendum, the UK Parliament passed the 1998 Scotland Act, which was given Royal Assent on 19 November 1998. The first members of Scottish Parliament (MSPs) were elected on 6 May 1999, and the Queen formally opened the Scottish Parliament on 1 July 1999, at which time it took up its full powers.

Under the terms of the 1998 Scotland Act, the Scottish Parliament has the authority to pass laws that affect Scotland on a range of issues. These issues are known as 'devolved matters', as power in these matters has been transferred (or 'devolved') from a national body (the UK Parliament at Westminster) to regional bodies (the Scottish Parliament, the National Assembly for Wales, and the Northern Ireland Assembly). Education, Agriculture, Justice, and Health (including NHS issues in Scotland) are among the issues devolved to the Scottish Parliament. The Scottish Parliament also has the power to set the basic rate of income tax, as high as 3 pence to the pound.

The 1998 Scotland Act also provides for 'reserved matters', which Scots must take up through their MPs at Westminster rather than through their MSPs. Such reserved matters, on which the Scottish Parliament cannot pass legislation, include Foreign Affairs, Defence, and National Security.

In Scottish Parliamentary elections, each voter has two votes: one vote for the MSP for their local constituency, and one vote for the candidate or party to represent their Scottish Parliamentary Region. There are 73 local constituencies, and 8 Scottish Parliamentary Regions; each local constituency is represented by one local MSP, and each region is represented by 7 regional MSPs.

These local and regional MSPs account for the total membership of the Scottish Parliament. Thus, every Scotsman or Scotswoman is represented by a total of 8 MSPs (1 local and 7 regional).

1. In the 1997 referendum, more voters in Dumfries & Galloway were in favour of a Scottish Parliament than were in favour of tax-varying powers for a Scottish Parliament.

A. True
B. False
C. Can't tell

2. The Scottish Parliament can raise the basic rate of income tax by 3 pence to the pound.

A. True
B. False
C. Can't tell

3. NHS issues in Wales are among the issues devolved to the National Assembly for Wales.

A. True
B. False
C. Can't tell

4. There are a total of 129 MSPs in the Scottish Parliament.

A. True
B. False
C. Can't tell

Practice questions provided by Kaplan Test Prep, a leading provider of preparation for the UKCAT and BMAT.
See www.kaptest.co.uk/ukcat/practice-questions, then enter your details to receive your Free UKCAT Starter Kit via email.

Verbal Reasoning Practice Questions - Answers

1. (A)
2. (B)
3. (C)
4. (A)

Answer explanations for each practice question can be found in Kaplan's Free UKCAT Starter Kit using the above link.

Quantitative Reasoning

The Quantitative Reasoning test is designed to see if you can solve problems using numerical skills. The test requires you to have good maths skills to at least GCSE level. That is not the main point of this test, however; it is more a problem-solving exercise in terms of taking information and manipulating it with calculations and ratios. As doctors are always using data, it is necessary to test this faculty. From drug calculations to medical research, applicants need to be able to show they have the ability to cope and can respond to different scenarios. You will be extracting information from tables, charts and graphs. There will be four items that relate to that data set with five answers to choose from. What you need to do is choose which is the best option.

Sample questions are provided on the following pages. It is a practice-driven section and, as with maths, the more practice you do, the more familiar you will be with answering the questions.

UKCAT Quantitative Reasoning: Section Summary

Number of scenarios: 9

Number of questions in each scenario: 4. These scenarios may be made up of charts, graphs, shapes or tables and you will have to choose between five answers. A calculator is allowed, though try not to use it all the time as it will slow you down and that is not the emphasis of the test. The UKCAT website quotes that this section, 'is less to do with numerical facility and more to do with problem solving.' Not being as strong in maths is not a factor therefore in this test; it is about strategy and thinking beyond the question.

UKCAT Quantitative Reasoning Practice Questions

Subtest length: 36 questions (9 sets of 4 questions)
Subtest timing: 24 minutes (2 minutes per set)
Sample length: 4 questions
Sample timing: 2 minutes

The total cost of hiring certain types of helicopters for certain numbers of hours is given in the table. Total cost equals the deposit plus the hourly rate per hour for the number of hours required. Some information has been omitted from the table.

Type	Hours	Deposit	Hourly Rate	Total Cost
A	3	£120	£225	£795
B	5	£300	—	£2,500
C	6	—	£495	£3,300
D	7	£575	£525	—
E	10	—	£575	£6,750

1. Andre's total cost of hiring a Type D helicopter was £2,675. What was the total time (in hours) for which he hired the helicopter?

A. 2

B. 3

C. 4

D. 5

E. 6

2. If the deposit for Type E helicopters increases by 30% on Saturdays, what is the total cost of hiring a Type E helicopter for 3 hours on a Saturday?

A. £1,914.00

B. £2,322.50

C. £2,602.50

D. £3,025.00

E. £3,600.00

3. Rupali hired a Type B helicopter for 2 hours on Thursday and a Type A helicopter for 6 hours on Friday. By how much does Rupali's total cost of renting a helicopter increase from Thursday to Friday?

A. 14.36%

B. 24.58%

C. 34.75%

D. 44.86%

E. 54.95%

4. The total cost of hiring a Type F helicopter is £1430 per hour. If Type F helicopters have the same deposit as Type C helicopters, what is the ratio of the hourly rate for a Type C helicopter to the hourly rate for a Type F helicopter?

A. 9:20

B. 12:25

C. 21:40

D. 15:26

E. 9:14

Practice questions provided by Kaplan Test Prep, a leading provider of preparation for the UKCAT and BMAT. See www.kaptest.co.uk/ukcat/practice-questions, then enter your details to receive your Free UKCAT Starter Kit via email.

Quantitative Reasoning Practice Questions - Answers

1. (C)
2. (D)
3. (B)
4. (A)

Answer explanations for each practice question can be found in
Kaplan's Free UKCAT Starter Kit using the above link.

Abstract Reasoning

Abstract Reasoning is designed to assess whether you can look at abstract shapes and then identify patterns, whilst ignoring the irrelevant material to avoid arriving at the wrong conclusion. What this test aims to do is test whether you are able to change your stance, be critical in your evaluations and create a hypothesis through inquiry. Patients often give doctors numerous symptoms that doctors have to work through to work out what is relevant and what is not in order to arrive at a diagnosis. Doctors therefore have to use their judgement, as patients are not always accurate in the information they provide.

In the UKCAT test, you may see one of four items.

- **Type 1:** two sets of shapes labelled 'Set A' and 'Set B'. From a test shape, you need to decide which set the shape belongs to, or neither.
- **Type 2:** From a series of shapes, you need to select the next shape in the series.
- **Type 3:** A statement will be given about a group of shapes and you then need to conclude which shape would complete the statement.
- **Type 4:** Two sets of shapes will be given to you labelled 'Set A' and 'Set B' and you need to decide from four options which belongs to Set A or Set B.

UKCAT Abstract Reasoning Practice Questions

Subtest length: 55 questions (11 sets of 5 questions)
Subtest timing: 13 minutes (1 minute per set)
Sample length: 5 questions
Sample timing: 1 minute

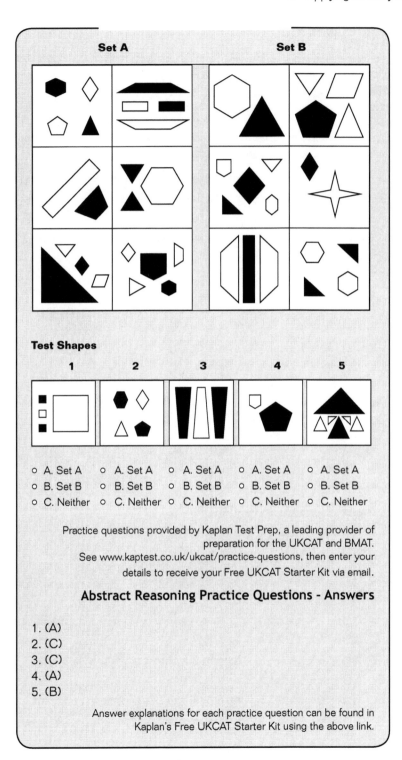

Test Shapes

Practice questions provided by Kaplan Test Prep, a leading provider of preparation for the UKCAT and BMAT.
See www.kaptest.co.uk/ukcat/practice-questions, then enter your details to receive your Free UKCAT Starter Kit via email.

Abstract Reasoning Practice Questions - Answers

1. (A)
2. (C)
3. (C)
4. (A)
5. (B)

Answer explanations for each practice question can be found in Kaplan's Free UKCAT Starter Kit using the above link.

Decision Making

This test assesses a candidate's ability to apply logic to reach a decision or conclusion, evaluate arguments and analyse statistical information. In 2016, Decision Making did not form part of a candidate's overall test score; however, that is no longer the case and universities are using this section as part of a candidate's score. For 2019 entry, you should make sure to check individual university websites for the most up-to-date information on UKCAT test requirements.

UKCAT Decision Making Practice Questions

Subtest length: 29 questions (individual items, rather than sets)
Subtest timing: 31 minutes (1 minute per question)
Sample length: 3 questions
Sample timing: 3 minutes

A queue at a corner shop consists of four people: Hamza, Iris, Johnny and Kenzie. Each person is buying a different item, including drinks (milk, wine) and snacks (ice cream, biscuits).

The person buying biscuits is standing somewhere between Hamza and the person buying wine.

Iris isn't buying a drink.

Johnny is standing directly behind the person buying milk.

Kenzie isn't at the front of the queue.

1. Which of the following must be true?

A. Hamza is buying ice cream.

B. Iris is standing between Hamza and Johnny.

C. Johnny is buying biscuits.

D. Kenzie is standing directly behind Iris.

2. Should it be illegal to eat any meat from animals or any animal products, like milk or eggs?

A. Yes, because there are health risks associated with eating too much red meat.

B. Yes, because we are running out of resources to support the meat demands of our rapidly growing population.

C. No, because there are some essential nutrients that are difficult to obtain in sufficient quantity without eating meat or animal products.

D. No, because it is not the role of government to pass laws affecting the food supply.

---

3. All my books are novels. Some of your books are non-fiction, but none of your books are biographies. This book is either yours or mine.

Place 'Yes' if the conclusion does follow. Place 'No' if the conclusion does not follow.

This book is a biography.	
This book is not non-fiction.	
If this book is mine, it is a novel.	
If this book is not yours, it could be a biography.	
If this book is not mine, it is not a biography.	

Practice questions provided by Kaplan Test Prep, a leading provider of preparation for the UKCAT and BMAT. See www.kaptest.co.uk/ukcat/practice-questions, then enter your details to receive your Free UKCAT Starter Kit via email.

Decision Making Practice Questions - Answers

1. (D)
2. (C)
3. NO; NO; YES; NO; YES

Answer explanations for each practice question can be found in Kaplan's Free UKCAT Starter Kit using the above link.

Situational Judgement

The Situational Judgement Test is designed to measure how you deal with real-world situations and whether you can identify critical factors and apply appropriate behaviour in the handling of them. What it is ultimately measuring is the level of integrity and perspective you will bring to the profession and whether you are able to work in a multi-disciplinary team.

You will be presented with different scenarios and each one will have different actions that you could take, with varying considerations. There is no expectation that you will have the procedural knowledge to answer these.

In the first set of questions, you have to determine the 'appropriateness' of the options in the given scenario. You will be given the following four options to give as your response.

1. **A very appropriate thing to do:** you should give this answer if it addresses at least one aspect of the scenario; it does not have to be all aspects.
2. **Appropriate, but not ideal:** you should give this answer if it was not an ideal solution, though it could be done, despite not being best practice.
3. **Inappropriate, but not awful:** you should give this answer if it should not be done, though it would not be considered terrible.
4. **A very inappropriate thing to do:** you should give this answer if you should definitely not do this.

In giving a response (i.e. 1–4), always remember that it might not be the only course of action and you should not consider it as such.

In the second set, you need to rate the 'importance' of a number of choices regarding a given scenario. You will be given the following four options to give as your response.

1. **Very important:** you would give this answer if this is vital to take into account.
2. **Important:** you would give this answer if it was important but not vital to take into account.
3. **Of minor importance:** you would give this answer if you should take it into account but it would not matter if it was not considered.
4. **Not important at all:** you would give this answer if you should definitely not be taking this information into account.

UKCAT Situational Judgement Practice Questions

Subtest length: 20 scenarios, 2 to 5 questions each (69 questions total)
Subtest timing: 26 minutes (20–30 seconds per scenario, then 10–15 seconds per question)
Sample length: 4 questions
Sample timing: 1 minute

During a busy weekend on call, Jagdeep, a first year junior doctor, is called to see Mr Morley, an elderly patient on the ward, who is complaining of a headache. Jagdeep has never met Mr Morley before. On his arrival at the patient's bed, Mr Morley takes one look at Jagdeep and states that he does not look old enough to be a doctor. Mr Morley says he should send someone more qualified instead. Jagdeep knows his seniors are busy seeing sick patients on other wards, and Jagdeep has many other tasks he must complete before the end of his shift.

How **appropriate** are each of the following responses by **Jagdeep** in this situation?

1. Tell Mr Morley that he can examine him now or he will likely not be seen by another doctor for a few hours.

A. A very appropriate thing to do

B. Appropriate, but not ideal

C. Inappropriate, but not awful

D. A very inappropriate thing to do

2. Ask Mr Morley how old he thinks he is whilst having a read of his notes.

A. A very appropriate thing to do

B. Appropriate, but not ideal

C. Inappropriate, but not awful

D. A very inappropriate thing to do

3. Tell Mr Morley that he does not look his age either.

A. A very appropriate thing to do

B. Appropriate, but not ideal

C. Inappropriate, but not awful

D. A very inappropriate thing to do

4. Tell Mr Morley he will send another doctor to see him.

A. A very appropriate thing to do

B. Appropriate, but not ideal

C. Inappropriate, but not awful

D. A very inappropriate thing to do

Practice questions provided by Kaplan Test Prep,
a leading provider of preparation for the UKCAT and BMAT.
See www.kaptest.co.uk/ukcat/practice-questions, then enter your
details to receive your Free UKCAT Starter Kit via email.

Situational Judgement Practice Questions - Answers

1. (A)
2. (B)
3. (D)
4. (D)

Answer explanations for each practice question can be found in
Kaplan's Free UKCAT Starter Kit using the above link.

In 2018, depending on your UKCAT score, you could apply for the following universities:

Score: over 690

- University of Edinburgh
- King's College London
- Newcastle University
- University of St Andrews

Score: 660-690

- University of Aberdeen
- Barts and the London School of Medicine
- University of Dundee
- University of Exeter
- University of Glasgow
- University of Leicester
- University of Manchester
- University of Nottingham
- University of Sheffield
- University of Southampton

Score: 600-660

- UEA
- Hull York Medical School
- University of Liverpool
- University of Plymouth
- Queen's University Belfast
- St George's, University of London

Score: Under 600

- University of Birmingham
- University of Bristol
- Cardiff University
- Keele University

UKCAT fees

- Test taken in the EU between 3 July and 31 August: £65
- Test taken in the EU between 1 September and 3 October: £85
- Test taken outside the EU: £115

UKCAT SJTace

The Situational Judgement Test for Admission to Clinical Education is being taken up for 2018/19 by the universities of Dundee and St

Andrews for their Graduate Entry Medical programme. It is designed to select the candidates who they deem to have the right professional behaviours necessary to be successful in the medical profession. It is identical to the Situational Judgement Test in the standard UKCAT test.

BMAT (BioMedical Admissions Test)

The BMAT is a test to ensure effective selection of well-qualified students. At present, 16 medical schools use this test (as outlined in Table 5) though only the following eight are UK universities. This is a written test and is deemed a productive indicator of a student's likely result in their first year of undergraduate study.

Table 5 Medical schools requiring BMAT admissions test

Medical school	UCAS course code
Brighton and Sussex Medical School	A100
University of Cambridge	A100
Chiang Mai University	Doctor of Medicine
Chulalongkorn University	Doctor of Medicine
Imperial College London	A100, A109
Keele University (for international students)	A100, A104
Khon Kaen University	MD02 (Northeast Thailand applicants, MDX)
University of Lancaster	A100, A900
University of Leeds	A100
Lee Kong Chian Singapore	A100, B900, B9N2 MBBS
Mahidol University	Medicine
Universidad de Navarra	Medicine
University of Oxford	A100, A101
Srinakharinwirot University	A10S
Thammasat University: CICM and Dentistry	Doctor of Medicine
University College London	A100

All candidates applying to institutions or courses in Table 5 are required to take the BMAT. The test, which takes place in November (usually in your school), consists of three sections. For a higher fee, it is also possible to sit this test earlier (in September) at one of the 20 testing centres available; this enables you to submit your result with your UCAS form.

Sample questions for each section are included below, courtesy of Kaplan Test Prep.

1. **Aptitude and skills:** such as problem solving, understanding arguments, data analysis, critical thinking, logic and reasoning (60 minutes; 35 multiple-choice or short-answer questions). This tests generic skills that will be useful at undergraduate level. The test is split into three sections:

   i.   problem solving: testing your ability to select relevant information and identify analogous cases (marked out of 13)
   ii. understanding argument: seeing if you are able to identify reasons, assumptions and conclusions and detect flaws in problems (marked out of 10)
   iii. data analysis and inference: looking at whether you can understand verbal, statistical and graphical information (marked out of 12).

BMAT® Aptitude & Skills Practice Questions

Have a go at the below sample BMAT Aptitude and Skills practice questions, taken from the full set.

DIRECTIONS (for full test):

Answer every question. Points are awarded for correct answers only. There are no penalties for incorrect answers.

All questions are worth 1 mark.

3. Media coverage of organ donation has increased as the Government considers making the donor registry 'opt-out', rather than 'opt-in'. Every week, newspapers and TV reports are filled with grim stories and statistics of waiting lists and deaths of those waiting for a transplant. Regardless of any changes to legislation, the media could do more to increase organ donation at present. For example, the frequent news reports on the need for more donated organs rarely mention how, exactly, members of the public can 'opt-in' to the donor registry. This practice stands in stark contrast to the presentation of such stories in other countries, such as the USA and Canada, where stories on the need for more organ donors almost always end with contact details for joining the donor registry. Providing viewers with a phone number or website for joining the registry is seen as a public service, part of the media's responsibility in calling attention to such a problem.

Which of the following best summarises the main conclusion of the argument?

A It's easier to become an organ donor in the USA or Canada than in the UK.

B Sometimes the media can help to solve the problems it identifies.

C The Government wants to make organ donation compulsory.

D Many people die waiting for organs each year as there are too few donors opting-in to the registry.

E Everyone should be required to join the organ donor registry.

4. Shannon and Dave are hosting a dinner party for six friends. The surface of the dining table is circular, with chairs set out equal distances around its circumference, as shown below. Each chair is directly opposite one other chair.

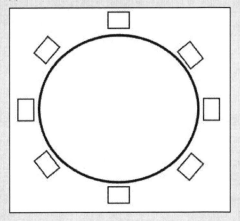

Dave prefers to sit directly opposite Shannon. Rachael and James are a couple, and prefer to sit next to each other. Ben fancies Lola, and he's a bit shy, so he prefers to sit directly opposite her. Dave and Shannon can't stand Patrick, whom Cindy is seeing, so neither of them will sit next to him.

If the seating plan meets everyone's preferences, what is the probability that Cindy will be seated directly opposite Rachael?

A 1/16

B 1/12

C 1/6

D 1/2

Practice questions provided by Kaplan Test Prep, a leading provider of preparation for the UKCAT and BMAT. See www.kaptest.co.uk/courses/uk-university/bmat/practice-questions/ bmat-prep-tools, then enter your details to receive your Free BMAT Starter Kit via email.

Answers

3. B

4. D

Answer explanations for each question can be found in Kaplan's Free BMAT Starter Kit using the above link.

2. **Scientific knowledge and applications:** the ability to apply scientific knowledge, from school science to maths (30 minutes; 27 multiple-choice or short-answer questions). You are tested on your core knowledge and whether you have the capacity to apply it – key for high level biomedical sciences. The questions you will have are related to material that would have been included 'in non-specialist school science and maths courses'. You therefore have to have a good level of understanding in these subjects. Questions are multiple-choice and calculators may not be used. Biology, chemistry and physics all carry eight marks each and maths carries six marks.

BMAT® Scientific Knowledge and Applications Practice Questions

Have a go at the below sample BMAT Scientific Knowledge and Applications practice questions, taken from the full set.

DIRECTIONS (for full test):

Answer every question. Points are awarded for correct answers only. There are no penalties for incorrect answers. All questions are worth 1 mark. Some questions have more than 1 correct answer. Read carefully to ensure that you select the appropriate number of answers. Calculators are not permitted during any portionof the test.

1. Haemophilia B (Christmas disease) is an X-linked recessive disorder. Both Jane's father and maternal grandfather suffer from Haemophilia B.

Which of Jane's relatives is neither a carrier of, nor suffers from, Christmas disease?

A Her sister

B Her father's monozygotic twin

C Her maternal uncle

D Her maternal aunt

E Her paternal grandmother

3. Three points in the (x , y) coordinate plane lie at:

(a, b)

(a+3$\sqrt{2}$, b)

(a+$\sqrt{2}$, b−4$\sqrt{2}$)

What is the area of the triangle described by these coordinates?

A $\sqrt{2}$

B 6

C 5$\sqrt{2}$

D 12

E 12$\sqrt{2}$

Practice questions provided by Kaplan Test Prep,
a leading provider of preparation for the UKCAT and BMAT.
See www.kaptest.co.uk/courses/uk-university/bmat/practice-questions/
bmat-prep-tools, then enter your details to receive your
Free BMAT Starter Kit via email.

Answers

1. C

3. D

Answer explanations for each question can be found in
Kaplan's Free BMAT Starter Kit using the above link.

3. **Writing task:** this tests your ability to select, develop and organise ideas and to communicate them in writing, concisely and effectively. You must complete one essay question from a choice of three, which requires you to construct an argument or a debate, analyse a statement or a similar yet equal-based task (30 minutes; one from a choice of three short essay questions). You have a choice from a selection of tasks and one must be selected. These will include brief questions based on topics of general and medical interest. The questions require you to explain or discuss the proposition's implications, propose counter arguments and identify resolutions. This is your opportunity to demonstrate effective written communication. Marks are awarded based on addressing the question in the way it is required, clarity of thought and concise expression.

BMAT® Writing Practice Questions

Time: 30 MINUTES

Have a go at the writing practice questions, taken from the full set. Here we show two of the four essay title options.

DIRECTIONS (for full test):

Answer only one task from the choice of four essay titles. You must write your answer by hand, and are limited to a space consisting of one side of A4. You are permitted to make any preparatory notes as needed, but time spent on such notes counts against the 30 minutes allowed for the essay. In this task, you are expected to show how well you can order and explore ideas, and convey these ideas in clear, effective writing. You may not use dictionaries or any other reference books or resources. Essays are assigned a numerical score. To achieve a top mark, you must address all aspects of the question and write compellingly with few errors in logic or in use of English.

1. A scientific man ought to have no wishes, no affections – a mere heart of stone. Charles Darwin

Write an essay in which you address the following points:

Why should those who practise science or medicine have 'no wishes, no affections'? What is the negative impact when scientists or doctors have 'hearts of stone'? How could a scientist or doctor best reconcile these competing concerns?

2. The greatest enemy of knowledge is not ignorance; it is the illusion of knowledge. Stephen Hawking

Write an essay in which you address the following points:

In science, how is the illusion of knowledge an enemy of knowledge? Can you argue that ignorance itself an enemy of knowledge? By what criteria could you assess the comparative impact of these two, to determine which is the greater enemy of scientific knowledge?

Practice questions provided by Kaplan Test Prep, a leading provider of preparation for the UKCAT and BMAT. See www.kaptest.co.uk/courses/uk-university/bmat/practice-questions/bmat-prep-tools, then enter your details to receive your Free BMAT Starter Kit via email.

Answer explanations for each question can be found in Kaplan's Free BMAT Starter Kit using the above link.

In Sections 1 and 2, points are scored on a nine-point scale to one decimal place. In Section 3, marks are awarded based on quality of content and quality of written English (A, B or C) and placed on a five-point scale out of 5. The written task is marked by the Admissions Testing Service.

The BMAT is a two-hour, pen-and-paper test. Unlike the UKCAT, you cannot use calculators or dictionaries, including bilingual dictionaries, in the exam.

Guidance on marks

- **Brighton and Sussex Medical School** score the BMAT out of 28: a total from all three elements and an extra five marks on the essay for good use of English language, making the essay very important to the process. Usually candidates with a score of 15.1 or higher are interviewed.
- **University of Oxford** looks for candidates achieving around 63% overall (Sections 1 and 2 are worth 40% each and Section 3 is worth 20%).
- **University of Cambridge** is more difficult to give exact guidance for as it applies a collegiate system (Oxford is centralised); however, the average offer holder achieves 6.1 (out of 9) in Section 1, 6.2 (out of 9) in Section 2 and around 3.3 (out of 5) in Section 3.
- **Imperial College London** is still the only university to have a cut-off score across three sections below which you will not be shortlisted. Section 1: 4.5 (out of 9), Section 2: 4.6 (out of 9) and Section 3: 2.5 (out of 5).
- **University of Leeds** took students last year whose scores ranged from 8.25 to 21.25 out of 23.
- **University of Lancaster** scores the BMAT out of 13, a total from all three elements, without the extra 5 marks on the essay for English applied by Brighton and Sussex Medical School. Usually candidates with a score of 10.5 or higher are interviewed (meaning you need to achieve, roughly, Section 1: 4.0, Section 2: 4.0 and Section 3: 2.5).
- **University College London** considers a good BMAT result helpful to your application though not the only factor. High scores for interview selection last year were Section 1: 5.3 (out of 9), Section 2: 5.3 (out of 9) and Section 3: around 3.3 (out of 5).

General hints

- Familiarity with the basic structure of the test is good preparation – however, it is not a test you can revise for.
- Do not waste your money paying for a tutor to help you learn for this; it is testing your ability.
- As with the UKCAT, the majority of candidates do not complete all sections in the test so don't worry if you don't. Ensure that you have tried the practice tests first so that you understand the timing of the test. Try to answer as many questions as you can but do not worry if you do not get to the end of each section.

- In sections 1 and 2, there is a point for each right answer, but no points are deducted for wrong answers.
- In section 3, each of the essays is double marked and there is a mark for the quality of written English presentation.
- Try your best to avoid leaving unanswered questions. Read the question thoroughly to try to work out what the possible answer could be by ruling out other answers.
- It might be obvious, but the best thing you can do is stay calm. If you have put in the time to practise beforehand, then you have prepared as best you can. Do not ruin your chances by letting nerves get in your way.

Dates

A list of important dates regarding the BMAT exam can be found at www.bmat.org.uk. For those students wishing to apply for entry in 2019 (based on 2017/18 entry timescale), the most important ones are as follows:

- registration opens: 3 July (September sitting) and 1 September (October/November sitting)
- registration deadline: 18 August (September sitting) and 1 October (October/November sitting)
- late registration deadline: 15 October
- takes place on: 9 September and 2 November
- results released: 23 November

Commitment

Have you shown a genuine interest in medicine?

This question has to be answered partly by your reference and partly by you in your personal statement but, before we go on, it's time for a bit of soul-searching in the form of a short test, found on the following page. Get a piece of paper and do this immediately, before you read on.

The *Getting into Medical School* genuine interest test

Answer all the questions truthfully.

- Do you regularly read the following for articles about medicine?

  o   Daily broadsheet newspapers
  o   *New Scientist*

- ○   *Student BMJ*
- ○   www.nhs.uk/Pages/HomePage.aspx
- Do you regularly watch medical dramas and current affairs programmes such as *Panorama* or *Newsnight*?
- Do you possess any books about the human body or medicine, or do you visit medical websites?
- Have you attended a first-aid course?
- Have you arranged a visit to your local GP?
- Have you arranged to visit your local hospital in order to see the work of doctors at first hand?
- What day of the week does your favourite newspaper publish a health section?
- Do you know how many different types of specialisms there are in medicine?
- Who is the Health Secretary in the UK?
- What do you know about the NHS?
- Do you know the main causes of death in this country?
- Do you know what the following stand for?

  - ○   GMC
  - ○   BMA
  - ○   NICE
  - ○   AIDS
  - ○   SARS
  - ○   MMR
  - ○   MRSA
  - ○   H5N1

You should have answered 'yes' to most of the first six questions and should have been able to give answers to the last six. A low score (mainly 'no' and 'don't know' answers) should make you ask yourself whether you really are sufficiently interested in medicine as a career. If you achieved a high score, you need to ensure that you communicate your interest in your UCAS application. The chapter will soon go on to explain how, but first a note about work experience and courses.

Have you done relevant work experience and courses?

It is always advisable to arrange your own work experience, and it is perfectly reasonable to use contacts, whether family members or friends, but medical schools will not want to see in your personal statement that you have shadowed a parent after they arranged the work experience for you. Organisational abilities are a vital component of becoming a doctor. This could be used as an important means of proving that you have the necessary skill set.

In addition to making brief visits to your local hospital and GP's surgery (which you should be able to arrange through your school or with the help of your parents), it is important to undertake a longer period of relevant work experience. If possible, try to get work experience that involves the gritty, unglamorous side of patient care. A week spent helping elderly and confused patients walk to the toilet is worth a month in the hospital laboratory helping the technicians carry out routine tests. Unfortunately, these hospital jobs are hard to get, and you may have to offer to work at weekends or at night. If that fails, you should try your local hospice or care home.

Hospices tend to be short of money because they are maintained by voluntary donations. They are usually happy to take on conscientious volunteers, and the work they do (caring for the terminally ill) is particularly appropriate. Remember that you are not only working in a hospital/ hospice in order to learn about medicine in action. You are also there to prove (to yourself as well as to the admissions tutors) that you have the dedication and stomach for what is often an unpleasant and upsetting work environment. You should be able to get the address of your nearest hospice from your GP's surgery or online.

TIP!

Because of health and safety regulations, it is not always possible to arrange work experience or voluntary work with GPs, in hospitals or in hospices. The medical schools' selectors are aware of this but they will expect you to have found alternatives.

Volunteer work with a local charity is a good way of demonstrating your commitment as well as giving you the opportunity to find out more about medicine. The CEO of a leading charity confirmed this to us in a recent talk, when he said:

> 'The purpose of the voluntary sector is to help people in need. However, we need help ourselves in order to survive as charities and continue to provide the support required by so many. Student volunteers are invaluable because they bring enthusiasm and purpose which the elderly respond to. Whilst these work experiences are good for their applications to medical school, I would advise very strongly that they investigate the nature of the charity before they embark on it because work experience is only truly relevant and productive when you can connect to the work and the cause, not simply be undertaking it for the sake of ticking boxes.'

Contact details for some of the respective charities can be found at the end of this book, although it is by no means exhaustive.

Any medical contact is better than none, so clerical work in a medical environment, work in a hospital magazine stall or voluntary work for a charity working in a medical-related area is better than no work experience at all. When you come to write the personal statement section of your UCAS application you will want to describe your practical experience of medicine in some detail. Say what you did, what you saw and what insights you gained from it. As always, include details that could provide the signpost to an interesting question in your interview.

For example, suppose you write: 'During the year that I worked on Sunday evenings at St Sebastian's Hospice, I saw a number of patients who were suffering from cancer and it was interesting to observe the treatment they received and watch its effects.' A generous interviewer will ask you about the management of cancer, and you have an opportunity to impress if you can explain the use of drugs, radiotherapy, diet, exercise, etc. The other benefit of work in a medical environment is that you may be able to make a good impression on the senior staff you have worked for. If they are prepared to write a brief reference and send it to your school, the teacher writing your reference will be able to quote from it.

Always keep a diary

During your work experience, keep a diary and write down what you see being done. At the time, you may think that you will remember what you saw, but it could be as long as 18 months between the work experience and an interview, and you will almost certainly forget vital details. Very often, applicants are asked at interview to expand on something interesting on their UCAS application. For example:

Interviewer: I see that you observed a kidney transplant. What does that involve?

Candidate: Er.

Interviewer: You probably weren't able to get up close to the surgery but can you talk me through the procedure and if you can, the reasons for it.

Candidate: Um.

Don't allow this to happen to you!

A much better answer should go something like this …

Interviewer: I see that you observed a kidney transplant. Why was that the recommended treatment for that patient?

Candidate: At Hospital GHI, this patient had been suffering from progressive kidney failure for many months. Without proper kidney function the body cannot remove toxins from the blood and regulate the ion and water concentration effectively. This can result in many problems like imbalance in sodium levels and high levels of urea in the blood.

Interviewer: What treatments are carried out for patients with these problems before we get to the stage of having to replace their kidney with a proper functioning one?

Candidate: Haemodialysis. This is when the blood is diverted from the body and put through a series of artificial membranes that act like the kidney would to filter out the wastes like urea and return the blood composition back to a level that allows the patient to have a decent quality of life. Some patients may have peritoneal dialysis when a catheter is inserted into their peritoneal cavity and dialysing fluid is passed through it. It remains there for a short time, about half an hour and this will allow the toxins to drain into it and then it is drained off. This allows patients to move around rather than in haemodialysis when they are connected up to a machine.

Interviewer: What are the main problems with a kidney transplant or any transplant for that matter?

Candidate: Tissue matching. That is the fact that body cells are covered in a set of proteins called antigens and these are specific for each person. If these do not match then the body recognises these as being foreign or what is called 'non-self' and initiates an immune response to destroy this tissue or organ and it is rejected. Finding organs that are significantly similar so as not to cause this reaction is very difficult and even if they do the patient is taking immunosuppressant drugs for the rest of their lives. This will make them more susceptible to certain types of infectious disease.

The only problem with work experience is that it can be hard to persuade members of a busy medical team to spend time explaining in detail what they are doing and why. MPW (Mander Portman Woodward school group, www.mpw.ac.uk/locations/london) and Medlink (https://medlink-uk.net) run courses for sixth-formers to help them understand the common areas of medicine and to link this theoretical knowledge to practical procedures.

Have you been involved in your local community?

A career in medicine involves serving the community, and you need to demonstrate that you have something of the dedication needed to be a good doctor. You may have been able to do this through voluntary jobs in hospitals or hospices. If not, you need to think about devoting a regular period each week to one of the charitable organisations that cares for those in need.

The number of organisations needing this help has increased following the government's decision to close some of the long-stay mental institutions and place the burden of caring for patients on local authorities. Your local social services department (its address should be in the phone book) will be able to give you information on this and other opportunities for voluntary work. Again, it is helpful to obtain brief references from the people you work for so that these can be included in what your teacher writes about you.

Making sure medicine is right for you

It is important to do your research into why medicine is indeed the right career choice for you. If you have chosen medicine for the wrong reasons, it is likely to come out at interview. There are short courses available to get a taste of the career, such as the PreMed Course, and others run by practising doctors at local hospitals who give an insight into medicine as a career. They do not intend to promote or glamorise medicine, but rather expose it as a profession. This might be an excellent way to assess your motivation at an early stage and also act as part of your work experience in medicine, which would be a good talking point at interview to justify your career choice. See www.premed.org.uk.

'All I really want to see is a student has a determination to succeed and one who has researched everything about the career path they are looking to undertake. Evidence is king, to misquote another saying. Remember that the person reading the personal statement has read hundreds, in some cases thousands of them before and therefore will be able to distinguish between what is real and what is embellished. Keep it interesting but above all else, keep it personal. Be truthful to why you want to study the course and what you have done about researching that. Remember the value of work experience is to educate and inform and confirm to you that this path is the one you want to take. Oh and don't swallow a thesaurus! Understand each word you write. Communication is the hallmark of a good doctor.'

Advice from an admissions tutor

Personal qualities

Have you demonstrated a range of interests?

Medical schools like to see applicants who have done more with their life than work for their A levels and watch TV. While the teacher writing your reference will probably refer to your outstanding achievements in his or her reference, you also need to say something about your achievements in your personal statement. Selectors like to read about achievements in sport and other outdoor activities, such as the Duke of Edinburgh's Award Scheme. Equally useful activities include Young Enterprise, charity work, public speaking, part-time jobs, art, music and drama.

Bear in mind that selectors will be asking themselves: 'Would this person be an asset to the medical school?' Put in enough detail and try to make it interesting to read. An important point to note though is that extra-curricular information must not take up more than about 25% of your personal statement, as the primary focus is on why you want to get in to medicine.

The key is to ensure that you are always relating your personal qualities and extra-curricular activities to your application, in order to show evidence of the attributes and skills needed to become a doctor. It needs to be relevant to the medical application, to demonstrate to admission tutors that you are the right sort of person for the university.

Here is an example of a good paragraph on interests for the personal statement section:

> *'I very much enjoy tennis and play in the school team and for Hampshire at under-18 level. This summer a local sports shop has sponsored me to attend a tennis camp in California. I worked at the Wimbledon championships in 2016. Doing so has placed the emphasis of team work and personal reliance on me. I have been playing the piano since the age of eight and took my Grade 7 exam recently; which I think demonstrates manual dexterity. At school, I play in the orchestra and in a very informal jazz band. Last year I started learning the trombone but I would not like anyone except my teacher to hear me playing! Music is a perfect way to relax, at the same time, it got me thinking about the link between music and medicine. The discipline and dedication of years of practice required in both is similar – not to mention the manual dexterity integral in each – but more so, looking into it, I have become fascinated by the link between the two, both from a therapeutic perspective – music therapy for example being a new technique designed to interact with patients – and a relaxation standpoint; anything from the music in a doctor's waiting room to the music playing in an operating room to calm the surgeon and help them focus. I like dancing and social events but my main form of relaxation is gardening. I have started a small business helping my neighbours to improve their gardens – which also brings in some extra money.'*

And here's how not to do it:

> 'I play tennis in competitions and the piano and trombone. I like
> gardening.'

But what if you aren't musical, can't play tennis and find geraniums
boring? It depends when you are reading this. Anyone with enough drive
to become a doctor can probably rustle up an interest or two in six
months. If you haven't even got that long, then it would be sensible to
devote most of your personal statement to your interest in medicine.

Have you contributed to school activities?

This is largely covered by the section on interests, but it is worth noting
that the selector is looking for someone who will contribute to the communal life of the medical school. If you have been involved in organising
things in your school, do remember to include the details. Don't forget
to say that you ran the school's fundraising barbecue or that you
organised a sponsored jog in aid of disabled children – if you did so.
Conversely, medical schools are less interested in applicants whose
activities are exclusively solitary or cannot take place in the medical
school environment. Don't expect to get much credit for:

> 'My main interest is going for long walks in desolate places by
> myself or in the company of my iPod.'

Have you any achievements or leadership experience
to your credit?

You should bear in mind that the selectors are looking for applicants
who stand out and who have done more with their lives than the absolute minimum. They are particularly attracted by excellence in any
sphere. Have you competed in any activity at a high level or received a
prize or other recognition for your achievements? Have you organised
and led any events or team games? Were you elected as class representative to the school council? If so, make sure that you include it in
your personal statement.

WARNING!

- Don't copy any of the paragraphs above on to your own UCAS
  application.
- Don't write anything that isn't true.
- Don't write anything you can't talk about at the interview.
- Avoid over-complicated, over-formal styles of writing. Read
  your personal statement out loud; if it doesn't sound like you
  speaking, rewrite it.

The UCAS application

'How important is the personal statement? It gets the foot in the door. Without a good personal statement, you may not progress to the other stages where you will shine.'

Dr Vicki Cooney; practising GP, London

You will receive advice from your school on how to complete a UCAS application, and you may also find it helpful to consult *How to Complete Your UCAS Application*, another title in this series (see page 195 for details). Some additional points that apply chiefly to medicine are set out below.

When the medical school receives your UCAS application, it will not be on its own but in a batch, possibly of many. The selectors will have to consider it, along with the rest, in between the demands of other aspects of their jobs. If your application is badly worded, uninteresting or lacking the things that the selector feels are important, it will be put on the 'reject without interview' pile. A typical medical school might receive well over a thousand applications. Table 1 on page 2 shows the number of applicants in the 2017–18 application cycle by geographic origin. The number of applicants at each university has to then be reduced to those who will be interviewed.

You can only be called for interview on the basis of your UCAS application. The selectors will not know about the things that you have forgotten to say, and they can get an impression of you only from what is in the application. We have come across too many good students who never got an interview simply because they did not think properly about their personal statement; they relied on their hope that the selectors would somehow see through the words and get an instinctive feeling about them.

The following sections will tell you more about what the selectors are looking for, and how you can avoid common mistakes. Before looking at how the selectors go about deciding whom to call to interview, there are a number of important things that you need to think about.

The personal statement

The most important part of your application is your personal statement, as this is your chance to show the university selectors three very important themes. These are:

- why you want to be a doctor
- what you have done to investigate the profession
- whether you are the right sort of person for their medical school (in other words, the personal qualities that make you an outstanding candidate).

Thus the personal statement is your opportunity to demonstrate to the selectors not only that you have researched medicine thoroughly, but that you also have the right personal qualities to succeed as a doctor.

Do not be tempted to write the statement in the sort of formal English that you find in, for example, job applications. Read through a draft of your statement and ask yourself the question 'Does it sound like me?' If not, rewrite it. Avoid phrases such as 'I was fortunate enough to be able to shadow a doctor' when you really just mean 'I shadowed a doctor' or 'I arranged to shadow a doctor'.

Another important consideration is the fact that your personal statement needs to be no more than 47 lines long or 4,000 characters (including spaces); this is a strict limit and so you need to ensure that you are as close to this as possible.

The personal statement is your opportunity to demonstrate to the selectors that you are fully committed to studying medicine and have the right motivation and personal qualities to do so successfully. A typical personal statement takes time and effort to get right; don't expect perfection after one draft.

Why medicine?

Your personal statement must, fundamentally, convince admissions tutors of your interest in following a career in medicine.

A high proportion of UCAS applications contain a sentence like 'From an early age I have wanted to be a doctor because it is the only career that combines my love of science with the chance to work with people.' Not only do admissions tutors get bored with reading this, but it is also clearly untrue: if you think about it, there are many careers that combine science and people, including teaching, pharmacy, physiotherapy and nursing.

However, the basic ideas behind this sentence may well apply to you. If so, you need to personalise it. You could mention an incident that first got you interested in medicine – a visit to your own doctor, a conversation with a family friend, or a lecture at school, for instance. You could write about your interest in human biology or a biology project that you undertook when you were younger to illustrate your interest in science, and you could give examples of how you like to work with others. The important thing is to back up your initial interest with your efforts to investigate the career.

Presentation

The vast majority of applications are completed electronically through the UCAS website using the Apply system. The online system has many useful built-in safety checks to ensure that you do not make mistakes.

Despite the help that the electronic version provides, it is still possible to create an unfavourable impression on the selectors through spelling mistakes, grammatical errors and unclear personal statements. In order to ensure that this does not happen, follow these tips.

- Read the instructions for each section of the application carefully before filling it in.
- Double-check all dates (when you joined and left schools, when you sat examinations), examination boards, GCSE grades and personal details (fee codes, residential status codes, disability codes).
- Plan your personal statement as you would an essay. Lay it out in a logical order. Make the sentences short and to the point. Split the section into paragraphs, covering each of the necessary topics (i.e. work experience, reasons for choice, interests and achievements). This will enable the selector to read and assess it quickly and easily.
- Ask your parents, or someone who is roughly the same age as the selectors (over 30), to cast a critical eye over your draft, and don't be too proud to make changes in the light of their advice.

TIP!

Keep a copy of your personal statement so that you can look at it when you prepare for the interview.

Five sample statements can be found below. They are all good examples of a personal statement made by a sixth-form student. Don't be put off by someone else's experiences. You have your own style and achievements, and what you have to do is write the statement in a manner that captures the reader's imagination and leaves them under no illusion that you are primarily focused on medicine as a vocation for life. Here, the examples demonstrate clarity and focus, and what comes through the most is the enthusiasm that the candidates have for medicine. These attributes will give an applicant an excellent chance of being called in for an interview and/or just being given an offer.

Example personal statement 1 (character count: 3,966)

I do not regret my unusual route; it is through studying architecture that I have become fascinated by medicine. Cities, like bodies, function through a range of systems operating at many scales, and are essentially spatial. They rely on material transport and homeostatic control, and are composed of highly specialised materials. The human body, at a fraction of the size, does this with an efficiency and elegance that I find compelling.

After graduating, I was awarded a research scholarship by UCL. I travelled to Colombia to study minimally invasive ways of developing slum settlements, and became interested in how specific architectural conditions could impact health. For example, due to space constraints, the residents all cooked on open fires indoors. The small homes were often filled with smoke, leading to high incidences of COPD and lung cancer. I looked at small-scale interventions, such as providing basic chimneys, that could significantly improve their quality of life.

Through studying A level Biology and Chemistry, I have been able to further my interest in medicine and medical technology. My thesis project at university looked at how cultured meat might be presented to the public in the future. I prototyped a range of synthesised biological materials and studied the laboratory production of muscle tissues and fats. Through studying genetics at A level, I have begun to understand how gene therapy could advance the use of tissue engineering in healthcare, for example, by reducing immune rejection. On a work experience placement at Great Ormond Street Hospital, I observed an ear reconstruction for a patient with microtia. Due to the rejection rate of artificial cartilage, the patient's lower ribs were used to form the structure of the ear. It was exciting to see how advances in tissue engineering could result in a far less invasive procedure.

Observing ward rounds and clinics, I quickly learnt the importance of interpersonal skills and clear communication. The doctors were able to broach sensitive topics with impressive care and professionalism and were articulate and exact when handing over patients. I was astonished by the number of staff involved in the operation of a hospital; team-work is evidently vital.

This is particularly true of interdisciplinary teams; with an increasing number of patients having multiple conditions, episodic treatment with 'siloed care', is becoming unfeasible. While volunteering at St Ann's, a school for children with special needs, I experienced the routine side of care. I was struck by the attentiveness of the staff, and found being able to gradually build relationships with those with mental disabilities challenging, but immensely rewarding. Volunteering at a drop-in centre for the homeless, I learnt the importance of establishing clear boundaries about what assistance could be provided, and was impressed by the way the staff could diffuse and manage aggressive situations.

I have spent the last year working for Hopkins Architects. Through client presentations, working to stringent deadlines, and coordinating information from specialists, I have been able to develop my professionalism, time management, and holistic thinking. My most testing experiences of architecture, however, were at university. 100 hour weeks were normal, and the working environment was intensely competitive. Team projects were stressful and emotionally charged. Leading teams of up to 20 people, I learnt to put aside quarrels and personal targets, instead focusing on the task at hand.

To relax, I practise mindfulness meditation and enjoy team-based endurance sports. At school I was an avid rower, and pursued this at a national level, as well as taking Duke of Edinburgh Gold.

The unsociable hours, bureaucracy and emotional demands of medicine do not deter me. It is a love of science, and a strong desire to place human well-being at the heart of what I do, that has led me to pursue this career.

Example personal statement 2 (character count: 3,967)

Medicine unites humanity against common foes and sees the frontiers of scientific research, philosophy and humane practice combine. This is what attracts me to it: the struggle to improve the world we live in.

One of these ruthless foes is cancer. Or would it be wiser to say cancers? Mukherjee explains that cancers are a heterogeneous family of diseases related by a common characteristic, the uncontrolled division of malignant cells precipitated by DNA mutations. I was intrigued to read of the myriad causes of cancers: Hepatitis B virus can cause liver cancer, exposure to radiation and sunlight various skin cancers and some breast cancers are even considered hereditary. This raises the question of whether Farber's 'universal cure' exists or whether the war on cancer requires an open-ended list of treatment strategies.

While shadowing a gastroenterologist at The Royal Marsden I witnessed a gynaecological surgeon open a woman's abdomen to treat cervical cancer which had metastasised to her bowel. Fascinated by the biology of cancer cells I read up on current oncological research. Could an implant loaded with the signalling molecule CCL2, which attracts certain immune cells and encourages cancer cells to follow, have identified the metastasis of the woman's cancer sooner? Or could adding microRNA molecules to cancerous cells turn them back into healthy tissues?

While shadowing a dermatologist at The Royal London I observed photodynamic therapy to treat a basal cell carcinoma on a patient's back. I learned about advances in immune therapy treatments for melanoma and how the drug ipilimumab blocks the inhibitory molecule CTLA4 on T cells, enhancing the immune system's anti-cancer response.

I also read that dogs could be used in cancer diagnosis, as they are thought to be able to smell the chemical changes in cancerous tissue, a certain wasp venom might kill cancerous cells and that Cuban researchers have developed Climavax, a cancer vaccine which encourages the immune system to attack a protein which fuels tumour growth.

At The Townhead Surgery I learned about antibiotic resistant bacteria, such as MRSA, and I have read that the GMC are considering censuring doctors who overprescribe antibiotics in an attempt to curb resistance. I was excited to learn that microorganisms in soil produce substances from which antibiotics can be developed and that scientists are harnessing the powers of these soil bacteria and fungi by growing them in labs between perforated membranes.

I have perceived the role healthcare plays in preserving the dignity of patients. Doctors must act with considerable empathy when assessing conditions such as psoriasis and the limitations of bowel control which can ensue after radiotherapy targeting prostrate cancer. In order to be a proficient doctor one must constantly educate oneself. In *The New Scientist* I have read about the flu virus and its evolving surface proteins which result in flu strains such as swine flu and avian flu. However, a universal flu vaccine is thought to be within reach after the discovery of proteins which don't evolve with the virus.

In 2013 I spent two weeks in Senegal working with Talibe children, helping to disinfect wounds and teaching English and French. I volunteer at St Joseph's Hospice which is teaching me skills of cooperation. I volunteered for two years at Steep Primary School as a classroom assistant. The experience taught me the benefits of patience and understanding and enhanced my skills of cooperation and communication.

In my final year at school I was headboy and part of a team communicating between the staff and student bodies which improved my leadership and teamwork skills. I have performed in a number of school plays and was a joint head of Senior Literary Society and Fairtrade Committee. I play the guitar and the trombone, enjoy team sports and played in the Bedales first teams for football and hockey. I now play for The East London Hockey Club.

Example personal statement 3 (character count: 3,985)

My journey to medical school has been long, carefully considered and slightly unusual. I read geophysics at the University of Durham and, although I enjoyed my studies, I became convinced that my vocation lay elsewhere. As a member of the Officer Training Corps, I trained with the Royal Army Medical Corps in trauma medicine in a hospital environment; the dynamic nature of medicine in a challenging environment hooked me. I also volunteered at Nightline, which introduced me to a different side of medicine. Acting as an emotional support for vulnerable people taught me the value of careful and proactive listening – vital for a doctor. The analytical and diagnostic skills developed at university, together with my rigorous science and military background, mean I believe I will cope well with the challenges of a medical degree and future career.

Since university, I have worked at a GP practice, both as a receptionist and as a clinical administrator. As the first point of contact between the practice and its patients, I would often be called upon to liaise with clinicians in both primary and secondary care in a variety of specialties. One example involved a patient who absconded from her psychiatric hospital and turned up at the front desk in a very distressed state. Having to take the patient aside, listen to her, calm her down and also liaise with a doctor in the building illustrated to me the importance of applying a delicate touch to a highly complex and stressful environment.

Through my work, I have been involved with the Planning all Care Together (PACT) programme – an initiative by Wandsworth CCG to combine community and social services in primary care to help patients suffering from chronic disease lead what is termed 'a more independent life'. Involvement included sitting in on and organising follow-up GP-led consultations. The project has taught me that even routine monitoring and procedures can be incredibly powerful, such as helping identify risk factors through blood test/lifestyle audits and ensuring people are allocated specialist care. I attended a conference, which discussed primary care-based anticoagulation therapy in atrial fibrillation sufferers, and learnt how primary care is now providing what was previously hospital-based treatment.

For over a year, I have been volunteering with St Mary's Hospital, Paddington in a respiratory ward, helping serve the patients their Sunday lunch and assisting the nursing staff each weekend. This not only gives me valuable clinical experience, but also emphasises how disabling a respiratory disorder can be and illustrates how resourceful and adaptable a doctor is required to be.

As the grandson of two cancer survivors, I was also keen to be involved in Macmillan Cancer Support. I have spent the last year involved with their 'Lewisham Buddies' program, a one-to-one weekly support meeting for cancer sufferers. I have experienced first-hand people fighting the disease and learnt the value to patients of gestures, even in a non-clinical setting.

My interest in the pathology of cancer, and its effect on people, led me to arrange a week's work experience in an Oncology Clinic in the Royal United Hospital (RUH), Bath, in which I saw the gruelling nature of its treatment. This led me to the subject of gene therapy, in particular, oncolytic virotherapy. I found a recent paper (*Nature*, 2012) on a phase 3 trial using T-VEC for metastatic melanoma of particular interest. I also experienced A&E and Orthopaedic clinics at the RUH, illustrating the demands of a junior doctor.

Alongside medicine, I have other interests; I coached football in my gap year, continuing this at university, in addition to boxing, and was an active member of the Durham Union. I feel that it would be a huge privilege to be able to pursue a career in medicine. I know that medicine is a demanding training and career, but my hands-on experience of working for the NHS has only strengthened my resolve to pursue a career in the field.

Example personal statement 4 (character count: 3,920)

My interest in medicine began with my father's diagnosis of haemochromatosis. It fascinated me how this could lead to many seemingly unrelated health issues. Having spent many hours visiting my father in hospital I was struck by the skill and compassion of his doctors in managing his complex health needs to give him the best quality of life. I can think of nothing more rewarding than being able to help people in this way.

Shadowing a consultant at the Royal Free Hospital allowed me to witness the value of teamwork as the MDT came together to discuss medical and social aspects of an asylum seeker's care. I felt the same empathy that the team demonstrated and saw how this enabled them to tailor his care. The value of good communication, leadership and teaching skills was evident as the consultant led a team of junior doctors to implement the planned care despite the staffing pressures they were under. At a GP placement I witnessed similar pressures and teamwork but saw the value of the closer relationships the GP had developed, allowing him to tease out an elderly cancer patient's concerns. During a Headstart course I enjoyed working as a team on a research task, discussing the science and ethics of our topic 'Three-Parent Babies'. On placement I discussed the consultant's academic medical career, and the ability to care for patients but at the same time carry out potentially groundbreaking research excites me.

Volunteering for a year at St Richard's Hospital allowed me to develop communication skills I had witnessed during placements. Empathising with patients allowed me to understand their anxiety and it was rewarding to offer comfort by listening to their concerns. These skills were challenged when I volunteered for Crisis At Christmas. I learnt the importance of being non-judgemental as many guests had dual diagnoses of mental health and substance abuse, either the cause or result of their homelessness, meaning they could be very volatile. I discovered extreme care was required in order to avoid unintended offence in unexpected situations such as simply serving tea. I secured a college travel scholarship to fund a trip to Africa. Climbing Kilimanjaro was one of the most challenging yet rewarding things I have ever done. Pushing myself to the limit mentally and physically taught me that I have the necessary resilience and determination to succeed in demanding situations, such as those experienced by junior doctors. Volunteering in Kenya, I enjoyed teaching and caring for HIV orphans. This required humour, patience and the ability to remain calm in hectic and stressful situations, employing skills I had witnessed during my placements. Seeing the kids' infectious smiles return after relatively simple treatments is my reason for returning during my gap year to run HIV outreach programmes, after I have completed my EPQ on the challenges of combating the spread of HIV in Western Kenya.

As Junior Captain of my athletics club I enjoyed developing my leadership skills in organising events. Through weekly coaching of juniors I have discovered a love of teaching and how satisfying it is seeing the kids achieve their goals. While academia is important to me, I am aware that medicine is a demanding career and of the need to maintain a work-life balance. Running plays a big part in my life. I ran the Brighton Half Marathon to raise £5,500 to help fund a medical centre in Kenya. I enjoy the team camaraderie of competing for my club, the social aspect of training with my friends and the stress relief of a solo run, and work this into my daily routine alongside my many other activities.

My experiences have allowed me to evaluate my desire to study medicine and appreciate the challenges involved. I believe I have the necessary intellect and personal qualities to succeed in a demanding but highly rewarding vocation, which will provide me with a lifetime of intellectual and personal challenges.

Example personal statement 5 (character count: 3,986)

Curiosity is imperative for the development of medicine: it acts much like a catalyst for the propulsion of new ideas into expert application. I feel that it is curiosity that has led me to pursue a medical career; this curiosity stems from both my scientific fascination and my ambition to help others through what I know and what I am determined to do.

Recently I have become excited by the potentials in genetic research. I completed a four-week MOOC, run by geneticists at St George's University, aiming to teach doctors about Genomics in Medicine. I also attended lectures at UCL about the prospects of recent genetics-related discoveries. I was particularly interested by the prospects of using GM crops to produce vaccines, evidenced most recently by the vaccine for the Ebola virus which can be produced by GM tobacco plants. To further my understanding of genetics I read Steve Jones' *In the Blood* and Richard Dawkins' *The Selfish Gene*. These books completely changed my perception on genetics – combining Dawkins' philosophical views and Jones' somewhat comical and factual interpretations. Currently I am researching a Nobel Prize-nominated development in genetic modification known as the CRISPR-Cas9 and its potential ethical issues.

Work experience in a multidisciplinary emergency response team taught me much about the Allied Health Professions. I was surprised by the diversity of the team, how each member could offer a different skill set and apply them critically. The team specialised in aiding elderly patients with recent engagements with hospitals. I learnt how proper documentation of each visit was vital for the well-being of patients through diagnosis and for future reference. I also volunteered in a care home, which gave me an insight into direct patient care. Communication with patients was often hard and so I tackled this partly by becoming a 'Dementia Friend' and by reading Oliver James' *Contented Dementia*, which helped me understand more about the condition and how to empathise more with the patients to support them better. This experience taught me a great deal about dealing with patients who often showed no clear indication of their needs.

In school I helped set up a medical society aimed at providing information to pupils thinking about careers in healthcare and medicine. I present discussions on ethical issues, carry out dissections, mock-up surgeries and practise using medical equipment. Through this club I myself have learnt much about the different areas of medicine as well as new and interesting recent developments while enjoying the benefits of teaching others.

Studying chemistry has helped me see how all elements are unique in offering characteristics of complex systems as they form shapes and bonds that contribute to individual processes within large-scale systems and how the human body can all be put down to the moving art of biochemistry. I was surprised at how such small changes to chemicals could have such drastic effects, such as with the optical isomerism of the drug Thalidomide; the original drug was a teratogen due to a slightly different arrangement of atoms in space that can only be seen by the effect of its rotation of plane polarised light.

Through the National Citizen Service, I was elected to run a social enterprise known as 'Free Spirit'. We worked with various charities to raise awareness about teenage mental health which resulted in us producing an effective and innovative product. We also carried out research on the physical as well as mental issues related to mental health after winning funding through a presentation to health professionals. We had an online campaign through social media to help refer teenagers to a specialised charity called 'Stem-4'. It was an unforgettable experience that provided me with skills in leadership and teamwork while working with new friends from across the country. I felt rewarded through helping others, which reinforced my ambitions to become a doctor.

WARNING!

Do not write any of the above passages in your personal statement, as admissions tutors are all too aware of the existence of this book. They also use plagiarism software to determine similarities between scripts. Ensure that your personal statement is not only personal to you, but also honest.

The reference

The reference will be written by a referee who could be your head-teacher, housemaster, personal tutor or director of studies. They will write about what an outstanding person you are and about your contribution to school life as well as your academic achievement (i.e. on target for at least three A grades at A level), and they will then also give reasons why you are suitable to study medicine. For them to say this it must of course be true, as referees have to be as honest as possible and they will accurately assess your character and potential to succeed at university. You must have demonstrated to your teachers and other members of staff that you have all the necessary qualities required to become a doctor. To start demonstrating this in your upper sixth year may well be too late – ideally these characteristics should have been evident over previous years.

To what extent does your referee support your application?

The vital importance of judicious grovelling to your referee and making sure that he or she knows all the good news about your work in hospitals and in the local community has already been explained. Remember that the teacher writing your reference will rely heavily on advice from other teachers too. They also need to be buttered up and helped to see you as a natural doctor. Come to school scrupulously clean and tidy. Work hard, look keen and make sure you talk about medicine in class. Ask questions that display your genuine interest in becoming a doctor or a particular topic, as well as thinking beyond the confines of the syllabus in class and ask intelligent, medicine-related questions such as those given below. Do not try and ask complicated medical questions for the sake of it; ask questions because you genuinely wish to know the answer and could carry on the conversation once given the answer.

- How effective is gene therapy in the treatment of cystic fibrosis?
- How does being obese actually contribute to suffering from type II diabetes?
- Is it because enzymes become denatured at over 45°C that patients suffering from heatstroke have to be cooled down quickly using ice?
- Could sex-linked diseases such as muscular dystrophy be avoided by screening the sperm to eliminate those containing the X chromosomes that carry the harmful recessive genes from an affected male?

Your friends may find all this nauseating – ignore them.

If your referee is approachable, you should be able to ask whether or not he or she feels able to support your application. In the unlikely case that he or she cannot recommend you, you should consider asking if another teacher could complete the application; clashes of personality do very occasionally occur and you must not let the medical schools receive a reference that damns you.

As part of the reference your referee will need to predict the grades that you are likely to achieve. The entry requirements of the medical schools are shown in Table 12 on pages 206–208. If you are predicted lower than the requirements it is almost certain that you will not be considered.

If you are a mature student or going through graduate entry, the referee could be a lecturer from your university who will provide the appropriate information.

Timing

The main UCAS submission period is from 6 September to 15 January, but medical applications have to be with UCAS by 15 October. Late applications are also permitted, although medical schools are not bound to consider them. It is recommended that students thoroughly check university websites to ensure that the given dates are correct. Remember that most referees take at least a week to consult the relevant teachers and compile a reference, so allow for that and aim to submit your application by 6 September unless there is a good reason for delaying.

The only convincing reason for delaying is that your teachers cannot predict high A level grades at the moment, but might be able to do so if they see high-quality work during the autumn term. If you are not on track for AAA by October, you still need to submit your application because, without an entry in the UCAS system, you cannot participate in Clearing.

Interviews usually take place between December and March of the academic year and so if you have not heard by January, it is not necessarily a negative situation.

What happens next and what to do about it

Once your reference has been submitted, a receipt will be sent to your school or college to acknowledge its arrival. Your application is then processed and UCAS will send you confirmation of your details. If you don't receive this, you should check with your referee that it has been correctly submitted. The confirmation will contain your application number, your details and the list of courses to which you have applied.

Check carefully to make sure that the details in your application have been saved to the UCAS system correctly. At the same time, make a note of your UCAS number – you will need to quote this when you contact the medical schools.

Now comes a period of waiting, which can be very unsettling but which must not distract you from your studies. Most medical schools decide whether or not they want to interview you within a month.

- If you have applied to one of those medical schools that do not interview A level candidates, the next communication you receive may be a notification from UCAS that you have been made a conditional offer.
- If one or more of the medical schools decides to interview you, your next letter will be an invitation to visit the school and attend an interview. (For advice on how to prepare for the interview, see Chapter 3.)
- If you are unlucky, the next correspondence you get from UCAS will contain the news that you have been rejected by one or more of

your chosen schools. Does a rejection mean it's time to relax on the A level work and dust off alternative plans? Should you be reading up on exactly what the four-year course in road resurfacing involves? No, you should not!

A rejection is a setback and it does make the path into medicine that bit steeper, but it isn't an excuse to give up. A rejection should act as a spur to work even harder because the grades you achieve at A level are now even more important. Don't give up and do turn to Chapter 5 to see what to do when you get your A level results.

Deferral of place

This is not a particularly advisable route in medicine, though not out of the question; the reason for this is that in such specialised subjects as biology, chemistry and mathematics, if you remain out of education for too long your scientific skill set will diminish. If you are going to apply to study medicine, you should expect to start as soon as possible, unless, and this is important, there is a good reason for you to make a deferral request. Bear in mind, universities are under no pressure to defer places as universities place a higher emphasis on places available for first-time applicants, except in extenuating circumstances. However, they do have roughly a 10% quota of students annually who will defer their places and they are sometimes happy to grant these requests if the student can prove they will be doing something worthwhile with their gap year. If there is a compelling reason, talk it through with them first to discuss your options there, as they will expect you to be undertaking something worthwhile in the intervening time.

Case study

Arthur Thomas is in his first year at University of Southampton, having completed his A levels in the first sitting. He received interviews and offers from more than one medical school and the deciding factor for him was the work experience opportunities.

'My first term at medical school was very enjoyable; however, it did take time to adapt to the new ways of life and learning. In my first full week, I attended a placement at a GP practice where I was taken to see a mother with a newborn baby to ask questions about birth and baby development. Having such early patient contact did surprise me but I was happy to engage in such a practical way of learning.

'The first term had been split into three main modules: foundations of medicine (anatomy and core sciences), a group project with a choice of topics, and clinical placements.

'There were a variety of lectures ranging from many different areas of medical and social sciences. Some lectures built upon concepts first learnt at A level and others seemed relatively new. I enjoyed learning about new medical developments and making links between different topic areas and clinical practice.

'I found learning anatomy fairly difficult; the way it was taught during the first term meant that I had to be very proactive and independent. I attended lab sessions where I worked within a small group to run through stations each lasting 15 minutes. We had certain tasks to do, such as identifying certain anatomical features and applying anatomy to clinical practice. To get the most out of each session, it was recommended to read the tasks beforehand and to study each area in some detail. As well as this, I had the opportunity to go back to stations that I may have struggled with.

'A few months into the course I was put on a placement in a maternity hospital where I observed and assisted wherever possible in a birth. I got to witness the intense emotions of the mother and her family, providing me with a greater sense of empathetic understanding, as well as the many roles within the multidisciplinary teams (MDTs) of the NHS. The experience was unforgettable and I felt honoured to have been given such a great opportunity.

'University life has so far treated me well. I have made friends from a range of courses and backgrounds. The medicine society has offered many social events and has its own buddy system whereby I have been assigned "medic parents" in the year above who have kindly offered to cook me meals and take me out every so often. There are plenty of societies to engage in, both within MedSoc (the medical students' society) and the students' union. The fresher events were a key part of my good experiences, with events such as balls and city nights out to act as key icebreakers for meeting new people.

'Studying at university may take a lot of adapting to for some students, but it is key to remember that many people are in the same boat and that universities accept each student for a reason, especially when they are studying a subject like medicine.'

3 | Mind over matter
The interview process

It's always difficult imagining what an interview is going to be like. All you can really expect to be predictable is the timeframe in which these interviews take place and this will traditionally be between December and March each academic cycle year. However, this doesn't mean that you shouldn't prepare. While it's very important to be natural, to ensure you don't reel off a list of pre-learned answers, you can still make sure you're prepared for some general questions and that you're able to give clear, well-worded answers and to act with real confidence.

Making your interview a success

If you are lucky enough to get an interview, you need to prepare thoroughly for it, as you will not be given a second chance if you do not perform well. As with most other activities, the more you practise, the better your chance of success. Interviews can be stressful and you will be nervous, and so practice interviews are an important part of your preparation.

In this chapter, we look at many of the common types of interview question and provide you with suggestions about how to approach them. We also give you advice on how to maintain some control over the interview and how to steer it to your strengths. You can then practise using the list of sample interview questions.

The questions that we look at in this chapter have all been asked at medical school interviews over recent years, and they have been provided by students who have been interviewed and by members of a number of medical school interview panels. You cannot prepare for the odd, unpredictable questions, but the interviewers are not trying to catch you out, and they can be relied on to ask some of the general questions that are discussed here.

For most questions, there are no 'correct' answers (but there are numerous 'incorrect' answers!) and, even if there were, you shouldn't try to memorise them and repeat them as you would lines in a theatre script. The purpose of presenting these questions, and some strategies for answering them, is to help you think about your answers before the interview and to enable you to put forward your own views clearly and with confidence.

When you have read through this section, and thought about the questions, arrange for someone to sit down with you and take you through the mock interview questions. (If you have the facilities, you will find it helpful to record the interview on video, for later analysis.) You might be interested in the views of four medical professionals, quoted in the *Student BMJ*, on the qualities that they look for. These views will not have changed; in fact, time and time again they are emphasised by professionals in this field.

> *'The medical schools are looking for well-rounded individuals that have interests in lots of different things, should be personable in order to be good with patients and have a good scientific knowledge which is par for the programme really. They are looking for lifelong learners, with a holistic approach to patients and able to maintain a good work-life balance. At times it can be a tough job and at times a very rewarding job and so they want people who can balance those stresses.'*
>
> Dr Vicki Cooney, GP and Medical Interview,
> Hammersmith and Fulham

> *'The innate characteristics of a good doctor are beneficence and the capacity to engage with the knowledge necessary for informed practice.'*
>
> Dr Allan Cumming, Associate Dean of Teaching,
> University of Edinburgh

> *'I think that you are born with some personal qualities, such as the ability to get on with people, to empathise with their distress, to inspire confidence in others, and to carry anxiety. Such qualities are very difficult to train into a person. A good doctor also needs knowledge and the experience of implementing that knowledge.'*
>
> Mike Shooter,
> President of the Royal College of Psychiatrists

> *'Medicine should always be regarded as a life commitment and not just a job. The demands put on you as a medical student and as a doctor will far exceed that of a standard job that some of your peers are able to land after just a few years of study and experience. It follows that making a commitment of this kind should not be taken lightly, especially when we see the strains and pressures put on the NHS and doctors which will ultimately lead to compromising patient care and safety. No one wants to be treated by an average doctor, in the same way as we would not want to be in a plane flown by an average pilot! So expect to be expected to be super human even when you know you aren't.*

'In other countries, such as the US, medical school is something you apply for after you have spent several years studying a degree or pre-med – I think this is a much wiser career choice as it will give you a few years to not only mature academically but to also establish your true calling. Studying medicine as a graduate may add on a few more years of study before you become a doctor, but it actually enhances your chances of getting the medical job you want – a reason so many medical students choose to intercalate. A doctor represents trust, integrity, compassion and someone who can make a significant difference to someone's life in an instant. Once you have honestly convinced yourself that you have indeed got what it takes, convincing admissions officers will be so much easier – learn to enjoy the pressure and remember that becoming a great doctor is a journey and not a target, so take your time.'

Kal Makwana, Executive Chairman of Medipathways

Finally, don't forget that medical school interviewers are busy people and they do not interview for the fun of it. Neither do they set out to humiliate you. They call you for interview because they want to offer you a place – make it easy for them to do so!

Typical interview questions and how to handle them

Why do you want to become a doctor?

The question that most interviewees dread! Answers that will turn your interviewers' stomachs and may lead to rejection include the following.

- I want to heal sick people.
- My father is a doctor and I want to be like him.
- The money's good and unemployment among doctors is low.
- The careers teacher told me to apply.
- It's glamorous.
- I want to join a respected profession, so it is either this or law.

Try the question now. Most sixth-formers find it quite hard to give an answer and are often not sure why they want to be a doctor. Often the reasons are lost in the mists of time and have simply been reinforced over the years.

The interviewers will be sympathetic, but they do require an answer that sounds convincing. There are four general strategies.

The story (option A)

You tell the interesting (and true) story of how you have always been interested in medicine, how you have made an effort to find out what is involved by visiting your local hospital, working with your GP, etc. and how this long-term and deep-seated interest has now become something of a passion. (Stand by for searching questions designed to check that you know what you are talking about!)

The story (option B)

You tell the interesting (and true) story of how you, or a close relative, suffered from an illness that brought you into contact with the medical profession. This experience made you think of becoming a doctor and, since then, you have made an effort to find out what is involved ... (as before).

The logical elimination of alternatives (option C)

In this approach you have analysed your career options and decided that you want to spend your life in a scientific environment (you have enjoyed science at school) but would find pure research too impersonal. Therefore the idea of a career that combines the excitement of scientific investigation with a great deal of human contact is attractive. Since discovering that medicine offers this combination, you have investigated it (and other alternatives) thoroughly (visits to hospitals, GPs, etc.) and have become passionately committed to your decision.

The problems with this approach are that:

- they will have heard it all before
- you will find it harder to convince them of your passion for medicine.

Fascination with people (option D)

Some applicants can honestly claim to have a real interest in people. Here's a test to see if you are one of them: you are waiting in the queue for a bus/train/supermarket checkout. Do you ignore the other people in the queue or do you start chatting to them? Win extra points if they spontaneously start chatting to you, and a bonus if, within five minutes, they have told you their life story. Applicants with this seemingly magical power to empathise with their fellow human beings do, if they have a matching interest in human biology, have a good claim to a place at medical school.

Answer with conviction

Whether you choose one of these strategies or one of your own, your answer must be well considered and convincing. Additionally, it should sound natural and not over-rehearsed. Bear in mind that most of your interviewers will be doctors, and they (hopefully) will have chosen medicine because they, like you, had a burning desire to do so. They will not expect you to be able to justify your choice by reasoned argument alone. Statements (as long as they are supported by evidence of practical research) such as 'and the more work I did at St James's, the more I realised that medicine is what I desperately want to do' are quite acceptable and far more convincing than saying 'medicine is the only career that combines science and the chance to work with people', because it isn't!

'The candidates who do best are those who are able to find something to be a good stress relief for them as the course can be quite overwhelming, from the interview process through to the job. We are looking for students who can balance their time so they do not burn out. In terms of an application, they need to be a reflective learner and to work out what kind of doctor they want to be, as this will affect the way they approach the degree. Also, there is no substitute to life experience, and we are looking for candidates who can bring themselves to both the interview and the job. Be confident and assured when you are at the interview; we are friendly and just want to get the best out of you, not make you so nervous you cannot even answer the questions. Try and enjoy the experience.'

Advice from an admissions tutor

What have you done to show your commitment to medicine and to the community?

This should tie in with your UCAS application. Your answer should demonstrate that you do have a genuine interest in helping others. Ideally, you will have a track record of regular visits to your local hospital or hospice, where you will have worked in the less attractive side of patient care (such as cleaning bedpans). Acceptable alternatives are regular visits to an elderly person to do their chores, or work with one of the charities that care for homeless people or other disadvantaged groups.

It isn't sufficient to have worked in a laboratory, out of sight of patients, or to have done so little work as to be trivial: 'I once walked around the ward of the local hospital – it was very nice.' You may find that an answer such as this leads the interviewer to ask: 'If you enjoyed working in the hospital so much, why don't you want to become a nurse?' This is a tough question. You need to indicate that, while you admire enormously the work that nurses do, you would like the challenge of diagnosis and of deciding what treatment should be given.

You also need to ask yourself why admissions tutors ask about work experience. Is it because they want you to demonstrate your commitment, or because they want to know whether you have stamina, a caring nature, communication skills and, above all, the interest necessary for a medical career? If it was simply a matter of ticking boxes, then they probably would not bother to ask you about it at the interview. They ask you questions because they want to know whether you were there in body only, or if you were genuinely engaged with what was happening around you.

Why have you applied to this medical school?

Don't say:

- it has a good reputation (all UK medical schools have good reputations)
- you have low entrance requirements
- my father studied here
- it is close to the city's nightclubs.

Some of the reasons that you might have are given below.

- **Talking to people.** You have made a thorough investigation of a number of the medical schools that you have considered, by talking to your teachers, doctors and medical students you encountered during your work experience, and current students. They have given you a good picture of what it would be like to study here and have all said that it would suit you perfectly.
- **The course.** You have read the course details and feel that it is structured in a way that suits your style of study and medical interests. You like the fact that it is integrated/traditional/PBL and that students are brought into contact with patients at an early date. Another related reason might be that you are attracted by the subject-based or systems-based teaching approach.
- **The open day.** You visited a number of medical schools' open days and this one was by far the most interesting and informative. While there, you talked to current medical students. You have spoken to the admissions tutor about your particular situation and asked their advice about suitable work experience, and he or she was particularly encouraging and helpful. You feel that the general atmosphere is one you would love to be part of.

Don't forget that all UK medical schools and university departments of medicine are well equipped and offer a high standard of teaching. It is therefore perfectly reasonable to say that, while you have no specific preference at this stage, you do have a great deal to give to any school that offers you a place. This answer will inevitably lead on to: 'Well, tell us what you do have to give.' That question is discussed on pages 97–98.

> 'Treat the additional questionnaire and any written correspondence as though they have the same importance as the exams and the aptitude tests. Any time the university asks for information, it is because they are seriously considering your application and therefore any half-hearted efforts will not be viewed favourably by the department. Simply call it, good practice in diligence for the profession.'
>
> Advice from an admissions tutor

Questions designed to assess your knowledge of medicine

No one expects you to know all about your future career before you start at medical school, but they do expect you to have made an effort to find out something about it. If you are really interested in medicine, you will have a reasonable idea of common illnesses and diseases, and you will be aware of topical issues. The questions aimed at testing your knowledge of medicine divide into seven main areas:

1. the human body (and what can go wrong with it)
2. discussing major medical issues
3. the medical profession
4. the National Health Service and funding health
5. private medicine
6. ethical questions
7. other issues.

The human body (and what can go wrong with it)

The interviewers will expect you to be interested in medicine and to be aware of current problems and new treatments. In both cases the list is endless, but the following are some areas with which you should familiarise yourself.

Your area of interest

This is how the questions might go.

Interviewer: I am aware from your application that you shadowed a consultant on the Minor Injuries ward and that you were interested by the different types of cases that doctors regularly experienced there.

Candidate: Yes, it was interesting.

Interviewer: Any specific examples of any injuries that stood out?

Candidate: All of it really.

Interviewer: What was the principal role of the consultant and what was his routine?

Candidate: Bits and pieces really. He made lots of notes and spoke to his clinical team but I am not sure what about as it was impolite to ask.

Avoid this situation by preparing well in advance. Choose a relatively well-understood procedure, such as ultrasound scans or a body system such as the cardiovascular system. Then learn how it works and (particularly for interviews at Oxbridge) prepare for fundamental questions such as 'What is meant by myocardial infarction?' and questions about what can go wrong with the system – see below.

Your work experience

If you are able to arrange work experience in a medical environment, you will want to reference it in your personal statement, but make sure that you keep a diary and that you record not only what you saw, but also medical details of what was happening.

For example, note not only that a patient was brought into casualty but what the symptoms were, what the diagnosis was and what treatment was given. Here is an example of a bad answer.

> **Interviewer:** In your questionnaire, you talk about work experience at Great Ormond Street. Could you tell me something about what you did there?
>
> **Candidate:** I spent some time shadowing two different consultants and was able to meet many of the children there who were suffering from a variety of different illnesses. I learnt about certain medications and saw how the ward structure worked.

The problem here is that the interviewers are no clearer about your suitability for a career in medicine, only that you have a good memory. This approach is referred to by some admissions tutors as 'medical tourism'. Interviewers are looking for a genuine enthusiasm for medicine. They are not going to be impressed by a long list of hospital departments, treatments or illnesses unless they can see that your experience actually meant something to you on a personal level, and that you gained insights into the profession. Here is a better answer.

> **Candidate:** I was very fortunate to get to spend some time at Great Ormond Street Hospital, particularly as I have an interest in paediatrics in the future. The design of the structure there means that everyone is required to be multidisciplined, and I was enormously impressed by that. As hard as it was to see so many children with such different illnesses, the thing I took away most was the professionalism of the staff and how they worked with the children. It made me realise that you treat each patient group differently dependent on their age. There is a big sense of family at the hospital and the activities available for young children is inspiring. More than that, I will take away how much confidence is required

and how crucial it is to keep calm in the face of difficult circumstances. As one doctor said to me, 'you are human after all; however, the trick is to realise that if it clouds your judgement, you are not going to help the person that you are empathising with to the best of your ability.' I felt that advice was invaluable. I also gained a lot from seeing the practical application of some of the knowledge I had learnt in A level Biology, as I was able to understand when the doctors were discussing parts of the inner workings of the human body.

In this type of answer, your genuine enthusiasm, good observation and respect for the profession are all apparent.

'The purpose of the interview is not to intimidate you, it is to get you to tell us why this is what you want above all else and what you have learnt. If we invite you to interview, you need to remember that it is because you have already jumped over a number of hurdles where many will have stumbled, and you are being seriously considered for a place at the medical school. This should give you a certain amount of confidence and hopefully allow you to enjoy the experience. Remember to maintain eye contact and body language throughout the interview, if you don't know the answer you can ask for clarification, however, try to give it a go; we will re-direct your answer if we need to and, most importantly, stick to what you know and not what you have *not* done please. We enjoy the interview process as meeting so many candidates from different backgrounds is the best part of this job. If you have any questions in advance, do not hesitate to contact the Admissions department – we can be friendly, despite the myth.'

Advice from an admissions tutor

Discussing major medical issues

Keep a file of cuttings

Make sure that you read *New Scientist, Student BMJ* and, on a daily basis, a broadsheet newspaper that carries regular, high-quality medical reporting. The *Independent* has excellent coverage of current health issues, and the *Guardian*'s health section on Tuesdays is interesting and informative. Newspapers' websites often group articles thematically, which can save time. The Sunday broadsheets often contain comprehensive summaries of the week's top medical stories.

Fashionable illnesses or the disease du jour

At any one time, the media tend to concentrate on one or two 'fashionable' diseases. The papers fill their pages with news of the latest 'epidemic' and the general public is expected to react as if the great plague of 1665 were just round the corner. In reality, CJD and SARS resulted in very small numbers of deaths, and the same can be said of recent flu outbreaks, for example. The media encourage us to react emotionally rather than logically in matters concerning risk. They advise us to stop eating beef but not to stop driving our cars, even though around 2,000 people are killed in road accidents every year. Thus, it is good to be aware of this bias as universities may ask you at interviews why it is that despite higher death rates due to obesity or alcoholism, swine flu is getting 'all the attention'.

While these diseases tend to be trivial in terms of their effect, they are often interesting in scientific terms, and the fact that they are being discussed in the media makes it likely that they will come up at interview. The next few paragraphs discuss some examples of diseases and illnesses that have seemingly gained a certain momentum and critical mass in terms of numbers of people who are diagnosed as suffering from them and therefore have been brought into the public eye.

Glandular fever, known as infectious mononucleosis (mono), is often a common one amongst students at school. Transferred normally in saliva, it has gained the reputation of the 'kissing disease'. It is recognised by symptoms of a high temperature, sore throat, swollen glands and then fatigue. The symptoms can often pass within weeks but the fatigue can last for months after the illness has gone. There is no cure for glandular fever, although the symptoms can be reduced through treatment.

Chronic fatigue syndrome (CFS), also known as myalgic encephalomyelitis (ME), is characterised by long-term tiredness which does not disappear with sleep. At this time, there is no cure for CFS, and any drugs that are prescribed are done so to alleviate symptoms such as headaches rather than to treat the underlying condition.

It is estimated that around 250,000 people in the UK suffer from CFS. Around a quarter of these cases are serious enough to affect daily mobility and routine tasks. Some people simply get better over time and resume their normal lives, but others can remain affected throughout their lives. For more details, visit www.nhs.uk/Conditions.

Depression is also a reasonably common illness nowadays that you hear of among certain age groups. It gets a negative review at times from certain quarters; however, it is a genuine illness and affects a lot of people. Symptoms are often wide ranging as it can manifest itself in different ways and there is no one cure for it, with treatments often ranging from lifestyle changes to therapy and, in severe cases, medication.

Multiple chemical sensitivity describes allergy-like symptoms caused by exposure to a range of chemicals, including perfume, petrol or diesel fuels, smoke, and organic matter such as pollen or house-dust mites. Symptoms can include breathing difficulties, itchy eyes and skin, sore throats, headaches and even memory loss. The fact that there are so many varying symptoms and stimuli for the condition has led to scepticism about the real existence of the condition.

Lyme disease is an infection caused by a tick bite. The disease has a variety of symptoms, affecting the skin, heart, joints and nervous system. It is also known as borrelia or borreliosis. The disease is caused by the *Borrelia burgdorferi* microorganism, which is present on ticks that live on deer. The symptoms of the disease, which first manifests itself as a red spot caused by the tick bite, include headaches, muscle pain and swollen lymph glands, and eventually the nervous system is affected. The symptoms may be apparent days after the tick bite, but in some cases they only present themselves months or even years later.

These diseases and illnesses have become more well known in recent times and, as a result, have gained more media coverage. This has had the effect of causing greater concern to the general public, who may have been unaware of their existence otherwise.

An interviewer could decide to ask you about a particularly 'fashionable' illness such as flu, which has been reported heavily in the media, by saying: 'Why is flu again causing so much concern, when very few people have died from it?' It is important to know something about these illnesses (see Chapter 4 for information on swine flu, MRSA and HIV/ AIDS) but equally important to keep them in statistical proportion. For example, nearly 2 million people die as a result of contracting diarrhoeal infections each year, mostly the result of poor sanitation and infected water supplies, and over 5 million people die as a result of injury sustained in accidents or violence.

Obesity, smoking and loneliness are discussed later in the book.

The big killers

Diseases affecting the circulation of the blood (including heart disease) and cancer are the main causes of death in the UK. Make sure you know the factors that contribute to them and the strategies for prevention and treatment. You can read more about this in Chapter 4.

The global picture

You may well be asked about what is happening on a global scale. You should know about the biggest killers (infectious diseases and circulatory diseases), trends in population changes, the role of the World Health Organization (WHO), and the differences in medical treatments between developed and developing countries. You can read more about this in Chapter 4.

The Human Genome Project and gene therapy

You would be wise to familiarise yourself with the sequence of developments in the field of genetic research, starting with the discovery of the double helix structure of DNA by Crick and Watson in 1953. You should find out all that you can about:

- recombinant DNA technology (gene therapy, genetic engineering)
- genetic diagnosis (of particular interest to insurance companies)
- cloning
- stem cell research
- GM crops
- genetic enhancement of livestock
- 'pharming'.

Diet, exercise and the environment

The maintenance of health on a national scale isn't simply a matter of waiting until people get ill and then rushing in with surgery or medicine to cure them. There is good evidence that illness can be prevented by a sensible diet, not smoking, taking exercise and living in a healthy environment.

In this context, a healthy environment means one where food and water are uncontaminated by bacteria and living quarters are well ventilated, warm and dry. The huge advance in health and life expectancy since the middle of the nineteenth century owes much more to these factors than to the achievements of modern medicine.

However, with unhealthy eating habits and a sedentary lifestyle becoming more prevalent, one of the biggest problems developing in the UK today is obesity. It is becoming more and more of an issue and the associated problems are costing the NHS more and more money each year. For more information on this, see Chapter 4.

TIP!

When discussing medical topics, you will sound more convincing if you learn and use the correct terminology. For example, to a doctor, a patient doesn't turn up at the surgery with earache; they present with otitis. The best sources of correct terminology are medical textbooks, some of which are quite easy to understand (see Chapter 9).

The medical profession

The typical question is: 'What makes a good doctor?' Avoid answering: 'A caring and sympathetic nature.' If these really were the crucial qualities of a good doctor, there would be little point in going to medical school. Start by stressing the importance of the aspects that can be taught and, in particular, emphasise the technical qualities that a doctor needs: the ability to carry out a thorough examination, to diagnose accurately and quickly what is wrong, and the skill to choose and organise the correct treatment.

After this comes the ability to communicate effectively and sympathetically with the patient so that he or she can understand and participate in the treatment. The most important part of communication is listening. There is an old medical adage that if you listen to the patient for long enough he or she will give you the diagnosis.

Communication skills also have an important role to play in treatment – studies have shown that some patients get better more quickly when they feel involved and part of the medical team. The best way to answer a question about what qualities are necessary to be a successful doctor is to refer to your work experience. You could say: 'The ability to react quickly. For example, when I was shadowing Dr Ferguson at the Fletcher Memorial Hospital, I witnessed a case where ...'

The National Health Service and funding health

It is almost a no-brainer that you will receive a question on the NHS, particularly when it dominates so much of the news. Whether it be the closure of departments, the privatisation of services, the political battleground in inter-party politics or the junior doctors' strike, there is no week that goes by it seems without the media discussing the NHS in some way.

An application to a medical school is also an application for a job, and you should have taken the trouble to find out something about your likely future employer. You should be aware of the structure of the NHS and the role that clinical commissioning groups and foundation trusts play. You need to know about the recent changes in the way in which doctors are trained, and the career paths that are open to medical graduates. When you are doing your work experience, you should take every opportunity to discuss the problems in the NHS with the doctors whom you meet. They will be able to give you first-hand accounts of what is happening, and this is a very effective way of coping with questions on the NHS.

A typical interview question is: 'What are the main problems facing the NHS?' The most impressive way to answer this is to say something along the lines of: 'Well, when I was shadowing Dr Jones at St James's Hospital, we discussed this. In his opinion, they are ...'

This not only demonstrates that you were using your work experience to increase your awareness of the medical profession, but it also takes the pressure off you because you are not having to come up with your own views. However, be prepared to then discuss your answer in more depth.

You may find that you get questions about the junior doctors' strikes and the moral and ethical considerations of the decision to strike. You need to be prepared for any eventuality.

Private medicine

Another set of questions that needs careful thought concerns private medicine. Don't forget that many consultants have flourishing private practices and rely on private work for a major part of their income.

Equally, a number of doctors do not have the opportunity to practise privately and may resent a system that allows some consultants to earn money both within and outside the NHS.

Your best bet is to look at the philosophy behind private medicine, and you may care to argue as follows below.

Most people agree that if you are run over by a bus you should be taken to hospital and treated at the taxpayers' expense. In general, urgent treatment for serious and life-threatening conditions should be provided by the NHS and we should all chip in to pay for it. On the other hand, most of us would agree that someone who doesn't particularly care for the shape of their nose and who wants to change it by expensive plastic surgery should pay for the operation themselves. We can't ban cosmetic operations, so we are led to accept the right of private medicine to exist.

Having established these two extremes, one is left to argue about the point where the two systems meet. Should there be a firm dividing line or a fuzzy one where both the NHS and private medicine operate?

You could also point out that private medicine should not harm the NHS. For example, the NHS has a problem of waiting lists. If 10 people are standing in a queue for a bus, everyone benefits if four of those waiting jump into a taxi – providing, of course, that they don't persuade the bus driver to drive it!

Ethical questions

Medical ethics is a fascinating area of moral philosophy. You won't be expected to answer questions on the finer points but you could be asked about the issues raised below.

A patient who refuses treatment

You could be presented with a scenario, and asked what you would do in the situation. For example, you have to inform a patient that he has cancer. Without radiotherapy and chemotherapy his life expectancy is likely to be a matter of months. The patient tells you that he or she does not wish to be treated. What would you do if you were in this situation? The first thing to remember is that the interviewer is not asking you this question because he or she wants to know what the answer to this problem is. Questions of this nature are designed to see whether you can look at problems from different angles, weigh up arguments, use your knowledge of medical issues to come to a conclusion, and produce coherent and structured answers.

> **TIP!**
>
> You should remember that the interviewers are not interested in your opinions, but they are interested in whether you have understood the issues. A useful approach to this type of question is to:
>
> - explain the background to the question(s)
> - consider both sides of the argument
> - bring current issues or examples into your answer
> - only express a personal opinion at the very end.

A good technique for answering 'What would you do if you were a doctor and ...' questions is to start by discussing the information that you would need, or the questions that you might ask the patient. In the above example, you would ask these questions.

- How old is the patient?
- Does the patient have any other medical conditions that might affect his or her life expectancy?
- Why is the patient refusing the treatment?

The answer to these questions would then determine what you would do next. The patient could be refusing treatment for religious or moral reasons; it might simply be that he or she has heard stories about the side-effects of the treatment you have recommended. One possible route would be to give him or her contact details of a suitable support group, counselling service or information centre.

A classic case is someone who refuses a life-saving blood transfusion because it contravenes his or her religious beliefs. Fair enough, you may feel, but what if, on these grounds, a parent refuses to allow a baby's life to be saved by a transfusion? Similarly, in a well-publicised legal case, a woman refused to allow a caesarean delivery of her baby. The judge ruled that the wishes of the mother could be overruled. It is worth noting that the NHS (as a representative of the state) has no right to keep a patient in hospital against his or her will unless the medical team and relatives use the powers of the Mental Health Act.

> **TIP!**
>
> This example illustrates an effective general technique for answering difficult moral, ethical or legal questions. The interviewers are not particularly interested in your opinion, but they are interested in whether you have understood the issues. Always demonstrate this by explaining the extreme opposing views. Only then, and in a balanced and reasonable way, give your own opinion.

Euthanasia

To answer questions on euthanasia, start by making sure that you know the following correct terminology, and the law.

- **Suicide.** The act of killing oneself intentionally.
- **Physician-assisted suicide.** This involves a doctor intentionally giving a person advice on or the means to commit suicide. It describes situations where competent people want to kill themselves but lack either the means or the ability.
- **Euthanasia.** Euthanasia is a deliberate act of omission whose primary intention is to end another's life. Literally, it means a gentle or easy death, but it has come to signify a deliberate intervention with the intention to kill someone, often described as the 'mercy killing' of people in pain with terminal illnesses.
- **Double effect.** The principle of double effect provides the justification for the provision of medical treatment that has a negative effect, although the intention is to provide an overall positive effect. The principle permits an act that foreseeably has both good and bad effects, provided that the good effect is the reason for acting and is not caused by the bad. A common example is the provision of essential pain-relieving drugs in terminal care, at the risk of shortening life. Pain relief is the intention and outweighs the risk of shortening life.
- **Non-treatment.** Competent adults have the right to refuse any treatment, including life-prolonging procedures. The British Medical Association (BMA) does not consider valid treatment refusal by a patient to be suicide. Respecting a competent, informed patient's treatment refusal is not assisting suicide.
- **Withdrawing/withholding life-prolonging medical treatment.** Not all treatment with the potential to prolong life has to be provided in all circumstances, especially if its effect is seen as extending the dying process. Cardio-pulmonary resuscitation of a terminally ill cancer patient is an extreme example. In deciding which treatment should be offered, the expectation must be that the advantages outweigh the drawbacks for the individual patient.

Currently in the UK there is a ban on assisted suicide, with the crime considered to be manslaughter or murder, depending on the circumstances, which carries the maximum of a life sentence. The Tony Nicklinson case in March 2012 brought this law into question again and the courts found themselves in conflict with Parliament, which wished the case to be struck out on the grounds that the law on murder was absolute. However, the courts ruled that there was a case to answer. They forced prosecutors to clarify the law on assisted suicide. The case was granted a hearing in the courts later in the year. However, in October, the High Court rejected the 'right to die' appeal as it was concerned that this would set a precedent for murder. Campaigners continue to fight this ruling. There have been many cases since.

In 2013, the Court of Appeal and subsequently the Supreme Court rejected cases from Jane Nicklinson and Paul Lamb, though a third case was won in a case for a man known only as 'Martin'. As recent as 2014, however, there was a slight relaxing of the rules. The Director of Public Prosecutions, Alison Saunders, has said that 'those directly involved in a terminally ill patient's care are less likely to face criminal prosecution'. That said, MPs were allowed a free vote to debate changing the law towards assisted dying in the House of Commons in September 2015, concluding three to one against giving a second reading to a Bill to change the law. Assisted suicide remains a crime in the UK, punishable by up to 14 years in prison. This is a very contentious issue and, as you can imagine, even within the medical community opinion is divided. In short, it deliberates and questions the ethical conundrum of the right of the individual to 'die with dignity' when they so wish versus the argument that it goes against moral and religious teaching and that it is against God's law to take a life. The nature of this ethical dilemma is central to the role of a doctor, as some would argue further that it also goes against the moral duty of a doctor, which is to prolong life instead of shortening it. While not a legal case, in 2015 Simon Binner made the headlines as he posted on his LinkedIn page, details of his impending date of death and funeral, trying, in doing so, to bring the issue to the public conscious- ness again – to say that everyone has a choice (see Chapter 4).

As it is a controversial question, it is one that can often be asked at interviews. What must be remembered is that aside from your own beliefs, whether you do or don't support euthanasia, the de facto posi- tion in the UK is that assisted suicides are currently illegal. There is, however, a Swiss-based group, Dignitas, which to date has helped nearly 200 residents of Britain to commit suicide. This has been due to their extreme suffering, which has to be well proven and documented. Dignitas was organised in 1998 to help people with chronic diseases to die, honouring the wishes of the patient and those around them to end their suffering. There is currently nothing stopping UK nationals from travelling to Switzerland and being assisted to commit suicide, but, as the law stands, loved ones and friends may be prosecuted if they help. See Chapter 4 for more information.

So one of the key questions is: 'Could you withdraw treatment from a patient for whom the prognosis was very poor, who seemed to enjoy no quality of life and who was in great pain?' The answer to this question comes in two parts. In part one, you must recognise that a decision like this could not be taken without the benefit of full medical training and some experience, together with the advice of colleagues and the fullest consultation with the patient and his or her relations, as well as knowing your position according to the law. If, after that process, it was clear that life support should be withdrawn, then, and only then, would you take your decision. Part two involves convincing the panel that, having taken your decision, you would act on it.

Other issues

A good opening question is: 'Should smokers be treated on the NHS?' On the one hand, it is certainly true that smoking is a contributory factor in heart disease. Is it fair to expect the community as a whole to spend a great deal of money on, for example, coronary artery bypass surgery if the patient refuses to abandon behaviour that could jeopardise the long-term effectiveness of the operation? Conversely, one can argue that all citizens and certainly all taxpayers have the right to treatment, irrespective of their lifestyles. Further to this, one can argue that duty paid on cigarettes adds up to more than the cost of treatment.

Another series of questions recognises the fact that there is a limit to the resources available to the NHS and highlights the tough decisions that may need to be taken. The interviewer might refer to 'rationing of healthcare'. Suppose you have resources for one operation but two critically ill patients – how do you decide which one to save? Could you, for example, choose between someone who is morbidly obese and someone who had a heart attack while running a marathon? Or suppose that you can perform six hip replacement operations for the cost of one coronary artery bypass. Heart bypass operations save lives; hip replacements merely improve life. Which option should you go for? A similar thread would be based around education of people versus drug prescriptions.

Even more controversial issues surround surgery to change gender. Should these operations be performed when the money could be used to save, or at least prolong, life?

Events are constantly bringing fresh moral issues associated with medicine into the public arena. It is important that you read the papers and maintain an awareness of the current 'hot' issues. See Chapter 9 for further reading.

Questions aimed at finding out whether you will fit in

One of the reasons for interviewing you is to see whether you will fit successfully into both the medical school and the medical profession. The interviewers will try to find out if your views and approach to life are likely to make you an acceptable colleague in a profession that, to a great extent, depends on teamwork. This does not mean that they want to hear views identical to their own. On the contrary, they will welcome ideas that are refreshing and interesting. What they do not like to hear is arrogance, lies, bigotry or tabloid headlines.

These questions have another important purpose: to assess your ability to communicate in a friendly and effective way with strangers even when under pressure. This skill will be very important when you come to deal with patients.

You may be asked how you would deal with a minor road traffic accident. You are walking on a pavement when a cyclist is hit by the door of a car when the passenger is getting out. The cyclist immediately jumps up to confront the car passenger, and both people are very irate. You are the only person around. What do you do?

The type of answer the interviewer is looking for will include the following points.

- Try to defuse the situation; interrupt them by asking if either of them is injured. Tell them the priority is to deal with any injuries.
- Carry out basic first aid if required.
- Look out for any dangers. Is the bike in the middle of the road? Is the car door blocking any other vehicles? Is the situation safe? Should you call for help?
- Phone the emergency services if required.

Questions about your UCAS application

The personal statement section, in which you write about yourself, is a fertile area for questions; as explained earlier, you should have included some juicy morsels to attract the interviewers. The most successful interviews often revolve around some interesting or amusing topic that is fun to talk about and that makes you stand out from the crowd. The trouble is that you cannot invent such a topic – it really has to exist. Nevertheless, if you really have been involved in a campaign to save an obscure species of toad and can tell a couple of amusing stories about it (make them short), so much the better.

Even if your UCAS application seems, in retrospect, a bit dull, don't worry. Work out something interesting to say. Look at what you wrote and at all costs avoid the really major disasters; if you put that you like reading, for instance, make sure you can remember and talk intelligently about the last book you read.

Sometimes an amusing comment on your application followed up by a relaxed and articulate performance at the interview will do the trick. A good example is the comment that a student made about lasting only three days as a waitress during the summer holidays. She was able to tell a story about dropped food and dry-cleaning bills, and was offered a place. Of course, failing at a part-time job is going to be a funny story only if you are relaxed enough to make it amusing; by then you will have already proved to the interviewers that you are a strong candidate, for whom this incident was an anomaly.

Questions about your contribution to the life of the medical school

These questions can come in many forms but, once identified, they need to be tackled carefully. If you say you like social life, the selectors might worry that you won't pass your pre-clinical exams. On the other hand, if you say that you plan to spend all your time windsurfing, mountaineering or fishing, they'll see you as a loner.

The best approach is probably to say that you realise that medical school is hard work and that your main responsibility must be to pass your exams. After that, you could say that the medical school can only function as a community if the individuals involved are prepared to participate enthusiastically in as many of the extra-curricular activities as possible. Above all, try to talk about communal and team activities rather than more solitary pursuits.

You may find it helpful to know that, in one London medical school, the interviewers are told to ask themselves if the candidate has made good use of the opportunities available to them, and whether they have the personal qualities and interests appropriate to student life and a subsequent career in medicine. Poor communication skills, excessive shyness or lack of enthusiasm concern them, and will be taken into account when awarding scores.

Unpredictable questions

There are two types of unpredictable question: the nice and the nasty.

Nice questions

Nice questions are usually designed to test your communication skills and to assess your personality. A typical nice question would be: 'If you won 20 million pounds on the lottery, what would you do with it?'

- **Rule 1.** Don't relax! Your answer to this question needs to be as effective and articulate as any other and, while you should appear to be relaxed, you must not let your thinking or speech become sloppy.
- **Rule 2.** A nice question could also indicate that the interviewer has decided against you and simply wants to get through the allotted time as easily as possible. If you suspect that this is the case (possibly because you have said something that you now regret), this question provides an opportunity to redeem yourself. Try to steer the questions back to gritty, medical-related topics. See the advice on page 103.

In answering the above question, be very careful. Take time to think. You could approach it from a medical perspective and use the money to set up a foundation to research a particular disease or condition that means something to you. This is where background knowledge and previous reading can be brought into the interview. Talk about the disease and the point to which the current research has reached. This is a starting point for your investment and then your money could be used to develop medication, vaccinations or a cure or preventive measure.

Nasty questions

The 'interview nasties' are included either as a test of your reaction to pressure or in response to something you have said in answer to a previous question. Here are some examples.

- Why should we choose you rather than one of the other candidates we have interviewed today?
- How could you convince me that you would make a good doctor?

There are no right answers but there is a correct approach. Start by fixing the interviewer with a big smile, then distance the question from your own case.

Regarding the first question: there is one absolute mistake that you must not make. Never compare yourself with any other candidate. You have no real idea about the quality of the other students applying. It may well be that you think you have all the qualities required to make a first-class doctor, but so will they. You would not have made the interview stage if they did not. Concentrate on your qualities. Make sure you know which qualities you have mentioned on your personal statement. Do not just recall it word for word, and, whatever you do, do not say 'as I have written in my personal statement'. Know what you have written, be able to discuss it and use your work experience to justify your answer. You should have found out during your work experience which qualities you have or even how they have developed during it.

Make sure you practise these answers before you have an interview. Either arrange a practice interview at your school or find an institution that organises these events. The more practice you get at these sorts of questions the better you will become at providing an answer.

Another 'nasty' question – one that interviewees always fear – is being asked about something scientific or technical that they have never heard of. For example: 'What is the drug x used for?'

You are not expected to have the knowledge that a qualified doctor has and so you would only be asked this type of question if the drug in question had been in the news recently, or if you had mentioned something related to it in your personal statement. So your pre-interview preparation (making sure you are up to date with recent events and being familiar with your personal statement) will help you here.

Questions about your own academic performance

These are especially likely if you are retaking A levels (or have retaken them). The question will be: 'Why did you do so badly in your A levels?' Don't say 'I'm thick and lazy', however true you feel that is!

Another bad ploy is to blame your teachers. It is part of the unspoken freemasonry of teaching that no teacher likes to hear another teacher blamed for poor results. If, however, your teacher was absent for part of the course, it is perfectly acceptable to explain this. You should also explain any other extenuating circumstances such as illness or family problems, even if you believe them to have been included in the UCAS reference. Sadly, most applicants don't have one of these cast-iron excuses!

The best answer, if you can put your hand on your heart when you deliver it, is to say that you were so involved in other school activities (head of school, captain of cricket, rowing and athletics, chairman of the community action group and producer of the school play) that your work suffered. You can't really be blamed for getting the balance between work and your other activities a little bit skewed and, even if you don't have a really impressive list of other achievements, you should be able to construct an answer on this basis. You might also add that the set-back allowed you to analyse your time management skills, and that you now feel you are much more effective in your use of time.

You may also be asked how you expect to do in your A level exams. You need to show that you are working hard, enjoying the subjects and expect to achieve at least AAB (or more probably AAA – check Table 12 on pages 206–208 for admissions policies to the different medical schools).

MMIs

There is now a growing use of MMIs (Multiple Mini Interviews) at the application stage. The University of Leeds, for example, uses eight mini interviews, each lasting seven minutes in length, in order to get candidates to think on their feet.

The MMI stations are designed to assess the ability of candidates to apply their general knowledge in a series of different scenarios. They will very much test each student's communication skills and capacity for forming personal and reasoned opinions. The key is, there are no right answers and candidates should be prepared to balance answers and intuition over prior knowledge.

The stations have been carefully designed to assess the following attributes:

* compassion and empathy
* initiative and resilience
* interpersonal and communication skills
* organisational and problem-solving skills; decision making and critical thinking
* team working
* insight and integrity.

If you will be having an MMI then it would be a good idea to ask multiple members of staff at your school to ask you different questions and get you to think on your feet.

Sample MMI questions

Below are some sample MMI questions provided by www.multiplemini
interview.com:

Station #1

PROMPT (Read and consider for 2 minutes):

'Liberation Therapy' (LT), a vascular operation developed to potentially
cure multiple sclerosis (MS) in certain patients, has recently come
under very serious criticism – delaying its widespread use. Among other
experimental flaws, critics cite a small sample size in the original
evidence used to support LT. As a healthcare policy maker, your job is
to weigh the pros and cons in approving novel drugs and therapies.
Please discuss the issues you would consider during an approval
process for LT.

YOUR RESPONSE: (Speak for 8 minutes)

Station #2

PROMPT (Read and consider for 2 minutes):

You are on the committee for selecting a new Dean of Science. What
characteristics and/or qualities would you look for when selecting an
effective dean?

YOUR RESPONSE: (Speak for 8 minutes)

Station #3

PROMPT (Read and consider for 2 minutes):

Clostridium Difficile (C. difficile) is a type of bacteria that increases its
activity with most antibiotic use, and is therefore very difficult to treat.
Research shows that the most effective way to prevent the spread of
infection is frequent handwashing. However, many people have flat-out
refused to wash their hands in hospitals. The government is contemplating passing a policy to make it mandatory for people entering hospitals
to wash their hands or else risk being taken out of the building against
their will. Do you think the government should go ahead with this plan?
Consider and discuss the legal, ethical or practical problems that exist
for each action option and conclude with a persuasive argument
supporting your decision.

YOUR RESPONSE: (Speak for 8 minutes)

Source: www.multipleminiinterview.com
Reproduced with kind permission by Astroff Consultants Inc.,
2 St. Clair Avenue East, Suite 800, Toronto, Ontario Canada M4T 2T5
www.astroffconsultants.com

Your questions for the interviewers

At the end of the interview, the person chairing the panel may ask if you have any questions you would like to put to the interviewers. Bear in mind that the interviews are carefully timed, and that your attempts to impress the panel with 'clever' questions may do quite the opposite. The golden rule is: only ask a question if you are genuinely interested in the answer (which, of course, you were unable to find during your careful reading of the prospectus and website). Some medical schools will not allow you to ask questions of the interviewing panel. It is particularly true of MMIs. This is mainly because interviews are timed so precisely. Questions can be asked of other staff or current students during the time you are there, but not in the interview itself.

Questions to avoid

- What is the structure of the first year of the course?
- Will I be able to live in a hall of residence?
- When will I first have contact with patients?
- Can you tell me about the intercalated BSc option?

As well as being dull questions, the answers to these will be available in the prospectus and on the website, and you will show that you have obviously not done any serious research.

Questions you could ask

- I haven't studied physics at A level. Do you think I should go through some physics textbooks before the start of the course? (This shows that you are keen, and that you want to make sure that you can cope with the course. It will give them a chance to talk about the extra course they offer for non-physicists.)
- Do you think I should try to get more work experience before the start of the course? (Again, an indication of your keenness.)
- Earlier, I couldn't answer the question you asked me on why smoking causes coronary heart disease. What is the reason? (Something that you genuinely might want to know.)
- I'm really interested in the chance to do an intercalated BSc. At what point in the course do I get to choose the subject?
- When we come to choose where we will go for our elective, how much help do we get?
- How soon will you let me know if I have been successful or not?

End by saying: 'All of my questions have been answered by the prospectus and the students who showed me around the medical school. Thank you very much for an enjoyable day.' Big smile, shake hands and say goodbye.

How to structure the interview to your advantage

Having read this far you may well be asking yourself what to do if none of the questions discussed comes up. Some of them will. Furthermore, once the interviewers have asked one of the prepared questions, you should be able to lead them on to the others. This technique is very simple, and most interviewers are prepared to go along with it because it makes their job easier. All you have to do is insert a 'signpost' at the end of each answer.

Here is an example. At the end of your answer to why you want to be a doctor you could add: 'I realise, of course, that medicine is moving through a period of exciting challenges and advances.' Now stop and give the interviewer an 'over to you – I'm ready for the next question' look. Unless he or she is really trying to throw you off balance, the next question will be: 'What do you know about these advances?' Off you go with your answer, but at the end you tack on: 'Hand in hand with these technical changes have come changes in the administration of the NHS.' With luck, you'll get a question about the NHS that you can answer and end with a 'signpost' to medical ethics.

You can, if you wish, plan the whole interview so that each answer leads to a new question. The last answer can be linked to the first question so as to form a loop. The interviewers have only to ask one of the questions in the loop and you are off on a pre-planned track.

This idea never works perfectly, but it does enable you to maximise the amount of time you spend on prepared ground – time when, with luck, you'll be making a good impression. The disadvantage, of course, in having a set of prepared answers ready is that there is a temptation to pull one out of the hat regardless of what is actually being asked. The question 'Why do you want to be a doctor?' (which you might be expecting) requires a very different answer to the question 'Was there something that started your interest in being a doctor?'

One final piece of advice on interviews: keep your answers relatively short and to the point. Nothing is more depressing than an answer that rambles on. If you get a question you haven't prepared for, pause for thought, give it your best shot in a cheerful, positive voice and then be quiet!

Mock interview questions

As explained at the beginning of the chapter, interview technique can be improved with practice. You can use this section of the book as a source of mock interview questions. Your interviewer should ask supplementary questions as appropriate.

These generally fall into the following categories.

- **Background and motivation for medicine:** Can you tell us about any particular life experiences that you think may help or hinder you in a career in medicine?
- **Knowledge of the medical school and teaching methods:** What interests you about the curriculum at [medical school]? What previous experiences have you had of learning in a small group setting?
- **Depth and breadth of interest:** Do you read any medical publications?
- **Empathy:** Give an example of a situation where you have supported a friend in a difficult social circumstance. What issues did they face and how did you help them?
- **Teamwork:** Thinking about your membership of a team (in a work, sport, school or other setting), can you tell us about the most important contributions you made to the team?
- **Personal insight:** How do you think you will avoid problems of keeping up to date during a long career?
- **Understanding of the role of medicine in society:** What problems are there in the NHS other than the lack of funding?
- **Work experience:** What experiences have given you insight into the world of medicine? What have you learnt from these?
- **Tolerance of ambiguity and ethics:** Is it better to give healthcare or aid to impoverished countries?
- **Creativity, innovation and imagination:** Imagine a world in 200 years' time where doctors no longer exist. In what ways do you think they could be replaced?

Additional example questions

Questions appear from the following categories. Ask a family member, friend or teacher to work through them with you.

Background and motivation for medicine

- Tell us about yourself.
- Why do you want to be a doctor? What do you want to achieve in medicine?
- What aspect of healthcare attracts you to medicine?
- What steps have you taken to try to find out whether you really do want to become a doctor?
- What things do you think might make people inclined to drop out of medical training?
- Can you tell us about any particular life experiences that you think may help or hinder you in a career in medicine?

Knowledge of the medical school and teaching methods

- What interests you about the curriculum at [medical school]? What previous experiences have you had of learning in a small group setting?

- Tell us what attracts you most and least about [medical school].
- What do you know about PBL? Why do you want to come to a PBL medical school?
- What do you think are the advantages and disadvantages of a PBL course?
- Why do you think problem-based learning will suit you personally?
- What previous experiences have you had of learning in a small group setting?

Depth and breadth of interest

- Do you read any medical publications?
- What do you think was the greatest public health advance of the twentieth century?
- Can you describe an interesting place you have been to (not necessarily medical) and explain why it was so?
- If you had to have a gap year, and could go anywhere in the world or do anything, what would you choose to do, and why?
- How do you think the rise in information technology has influenced/will influence the practice of medicine?
- If you could invite three people, alive or dead, to dinner, who would they be?

Empathy

- Give an example of a situation where you have supported a friend in a difficult social circumstance. What issues did they face and how did you help them?
- What does the word empathy mean to you? How do you differentiate empathy from sympathy?
- Is it right for doctors to 'feel for their patients'?
- What do you guess an overweight person might feel and think after being told their arthritis is due to their weight?
- A friend has asked your advice on how to tell her parents that she intends to drop out of university and go off travelling. How would you respond?
- A friend tells you he feels bad because his family has always cheated to obtain extra benefits. How would you respond?

Team work

- Tell us about a team situation you have experienced. What did you learn about yourself and about successful team-working?
- When you think about yourself working as a doctor, who do you think will be the most important people in the team you will be working with?
- Who are the important members of a multi-disciplinary healthcare team? Why?
- Are you a leader or a follower?

- What are the advantages and disadvantages of being in a team? Do teams need leaders?
- What do you think is the role of humour in team working? Give an example.

Personal insight

- Give us an example of something about which you used to hold strong opinions, but have had to change your mind. What made you change? What do you think now?
- Have you ever been in a situation where you realise afterwards that what you said or did was wrong? What did you do about it? What should you have done?
- How do you think you will avoid problems of keeping up to date during a long career?
- What are your outside interests and hobbies? How do these complement you as a person? Which do you think you will continue at university?
- Tell us two personal qualities you have which would make you a good doctor, and two personal shortcomings which you think you would like to overcome as you become a doctor?
- Medical training is long and being a doctor can be stressful. Some doctors who qualify never practise. What makes you think you will stick to it?
- What do you think will be the most difficult things you might encounter during your training? How will you deal with them?

Understanding of the role of medicine in society

- What is wrong with the NHS?
- Would you argue that medicine is a science or an art, and why?
- Why do you think we hear so much about doctors and the NHS in the media today?
- In what ways do you think doctors can promote good health, other than direct treatment of illness?
- Do you think patients' treatments should be limited by the NHS budget or do they have the right to new therapies no matter what the cost?
- What do you understand by the term 'holistic' medicine? Do you think it falls within the remit of the NHS?

Work experience

- What experiences have given you insight into the world of medicine? What have you learnt from these?
- What aspect of your work experience did you find the most challenging, and why?
- Reflect on what you have seen of hospitals or a healthcare environment. What would you most like to organise differently, and why?

- What aspect of your work experience would you recommend to a friend thinking about medicine, and why?
- Thinking of your work experience, can you tell me about a difficult situation you have dealt with and what you learned from it?
- Have you visited any friends or family in hospital, or had work experience in a hospital? From these experiences, what did you see that you would like to change?

Tolerance of ambiguity and ethics

- Is it better to give healthcare or aid to impoverished countries?
- Should doctors have a role in contact sports such as boxing?
- Do you think doctors should ever go on strike?
- How do you think doctors should treat injury or illness due to self-harm, smoking or excess alcohol consumption?
- Female infertility treatment is expensive, has a very low success rate and is even less successful in smokers. To whom do you think it should be available?
- Would you prescribe the oral contraceptive pill to a 14-year-old girl who is sleeping with her boyfriend?

Creativity, innovation and imagination

- Imagine a world in 200 years' time where doctors no longer exist. In what ways do you think they could be replaced?
- You are holding a party on a medical theme. How would you make it memorable?
- Describe as many uses as you can for a mobile phone charger.
- How many different ways can you improve the process of selecting students for this medical school?
- Imagine you had six months with enough money and nothing you had to do. Tell us the most imaginative (and non-medical) way you'd spend the time.
- Your house catches fire in the night. You are told you can pick only one object to take with you when escaping. What would it be and why?

Points for the interviewer to assess

The following is a list of criteria that the admissions staff will be looking for when interviewing candidates to determine their suitability for the course.

- Did the candidate answer in a positive, open and friendly way, maintaining eye contact for most of the time?
- Was the candidate's posture such that you felt that he or she was alert, friendly and enthusiastic?
- Was the candidate's voice pitched correctly: neither too loud nor too soft and without traces of arrogance or complacency?

- Was the candidate free of irritating mannerisms?
- Did the candidate's performance reassure you enough not to terrify you at the prospect that he or she could be your doctor in a few years?

The panel

Most medical schools have so many candidates that they operate several interview panels in parallel. This means that your interview may not be chaired by the dean, but you will certainly have a senior member of the academic staff chairing the panel. He or she will normally be assisted by two or three others. Usually, there are representatives of the clinical and pre-clinical staff and there may be a medical student on the board too. Sometimes a local GP is invited to join the panel.

While you can expect the interviewers to be friendly, it is possible that one of them may use an aggressive approach. Don't be put off by this; it is a classic interview technique and will usually be balanced by a supportive member of the panel.

Questionnaires

A number of medical schools, in order to confirm the details provided, will send out a questionnaire in order to get more information before the interview so you need to be as descriptive as possible. Universities now mostly use the Situational Judgement Test (SJT) through the UKCAT instead of a written test specific to the university. A number of universities now use Multiple Mini Interviews (MMI) to assess candidates, so there will be exercises given during the day of the interview. Bear in mind that a candidate who performs well in the interview, displays the necessary academic and personal qualities and is genuinely suited to medicine is unlikely to be rejected on the basis of the written element.

Dress, posture and mannerisms

You should dress smartly for your interview, but you should also feel comfortable. You will not be able to relax if you feel over-formal. For men, a jacket with a clean shirt and tie is ideal. Women should avoid big earrings, plunging necklines and short skirts. Men should not wear earrings, white socks or loud ties, or have (visible) piercings. Avoid unconventional hairstyles: no Mohicans or skinheads.

Your aim must be to give an impression of good personal organisation and cleanliness. Make a particular point of your hair and fingernails – you never see a doctor with dirty fingernails. Always polish your shoes before an interview, as this type of detail will be noticed. Don't go in smelling strongly of aftershave, perfume or food. You will be invited to sit down, but don't fall back expansively into an armchair, cross your legs and press your fingertips together in an impersonation of Sherlock Holmes. Sit slightly forward in a way that allows you to be both comfortable and alert. Make sure that you arrive early and are well prepared for the interview.

Try to achieve eye contact with each member of the panel and, as much as possible, address your answer directly to the panel member who asked the question (glancing regularly at the others), not up in the air or to a piece of furniture. Most importantly, try to relax and enjoy the interview. This will help you to project an open, cheerful personality.

Finally, watch out for irritating mannerisms. These are easily checked if you videotape a mock interview. The interviewers will not listen to what you are saying if they are all watching to see when you are next going to scratch your left ear with your right thumb!

What happens next?

When you have left the room, the person chairing the interview panel will discuss your performance with the other members and will make a recommendation to the dean. The recommendation will be one of the following:

- accept
- discuss further/waiting list
- reject.

'Accept' means that you will receive a conditional or unconditional offer.

'Discuss further' means that you are borderline, and may or may not receive an offer, depending on the quality of the applicants seen by other interview panels. If, having been classified as 'discuss further', you have been unlucky and have received a rejection, the medical school may put you on an official or unofficial waiting list. The people on the waiting list are either re-contacted after students have nominated their choices and the picture has settled in May, or are the first to be considered in Clearing; although it should be said that you cannot rely on this possibility. In 2017, more universities – Bristol and Liverpool – followed St George's example and offered places in Clearing. If you have been rejected by all of the institutions you applied to, you can go through the UCAS Extra scheme, which gives you a chance to approach other universities. Details can be found on the UCAS website.

'Reject' means that you will not be made an offer. You may be luckier at one of the other medical schools to which you have applied.

The official notification of your fate will come to you from UCAS within a few weeks of the interview. If you have been rejected it is helpful to know whether you are on the waiting list and whether or not there is any point in applying again to that medical school.

Understandably, the staff will be reluctant to talk to you about your performance, but most medical schools will discuss your application with your UCAS referee if he or she calls them to ask what advice should now be given to you. It is well worth asking your referee to make that telephone call.

Case study

Tara struggled initially in her A levels; however, she took a re-assessment at the end of the first year and decided to move schools in order to realise her goal of studying medicine. She went from Cs and Ds, to A*A*A by the end of her A levels. She decided to take a year out in order to apply for medicine, as it was an easier conversation once the grades were achieved; her story should give anyone hope if they feel they are not on track.

'By the time I was sitting my GCSEs I knew I wanted to be a doctor. My GCSE results weren't great and were a bit of a shock to say the least. When I found out my results and that I'd got C in biology and physics and a D in chemistry I was devastated and thought my dream of medicine was over ... you need at least 10 A*s right?

'However, once I got over the initial shock, I knew that I (and other friends) should have achieved better and that the problems my school had with the science department probably hadn't helped. So, determined not to give up at the first hurdle I set about trying to persuade my new sixth form to allow me to still take chemistry and biology A levels. To say they were reluctant was an under-statement, but eventually they agreed to let me try. Something good that came out of my GCSE results was that I realised that I really couldn't rely solely on my teachers to provide me with every-thing I needed, and that I had to take responsibility for my own learning, which was a pretty useful lesson going into A levels.

'I worked really hard but had huge areas of knowledge missing that I hadn't been taught at GCSE, which wasn't a great start as I didn't know what was going on in half the lessons and had to catch up after. Unfortunately, most of my science teachers were really unhelpful, as I imagine they felt I had no place in their lessons, so I became really reluctant to admit if I didn't understand something. I sat AS exams and managed to achieve four Cs, which was ok but not great. My confidence was pretty low and I was questioning my ability to get the grades I needed. I decided that I couldn't spend another year in the same school as it would just knock me further, so I transferred to a sixth form with some amazing teachers who acted like they believed in me and totally rebuilt my confidence.

'I was advised, given my GCSE and AS results, that it might be better if I focus on getting good A level results, then take a gap year and apply with my results known. My parents were a little nervous in case I didn't get the grades I needed to get into medicine the first time round so I applied for biomedical science and was amazed to get five offers. I firmed a place at UCL for Applied Medical Sciences (AAB) – as I loved the uni and the course looked amazing – and insured St George's (BBB), as they offered a transfer to medicine scheme.

'I then spent the next nine months working my socks off and making sure I was ticking all the other boxes to get into medical school, by continuing with my work experience, volunteering and sport, running a half marathon for charity, etc. I did everything my teachers suggested and more, tackling every past exam paper at least three times!

'I knew that even if I managed to achieve great A level results, my GCSEs would potentially hold me back, so I read everything I could about the application process and what each individual medical school was looking for, attending their open days, talking to the admissions tutors to try and gauge their reactions. I emailed admissions departments and created a spreadsheet of each medical school, crossing off the ones where I felt I had no chance. Some came back and told me that it didn't matter if I got all A*s at A level and top marks in UKCAT, my application would be rejected instantly on the basis of my GCSE results so it was pointless to apply.

'On results day I was absolutely delighted that, with a lot of hard work and help from my amazing teachers, I achieved A*A*A in mathematics, chemistry and biology! I knew that I 100% wanted to go to a London medical school, and my dream was UCL who use a holistic approach; but they had been so vague when I spoke and emailed them, I really wasn't sure I had a chance.

'I'd won a travel award from my college so I spent the summer climbing Kilimanjaro, fundraising and volunteering at a centre for HIV orphans in Kenya, so by the time I came to write my personal statement it was a struggle to know what to include and what to leave out, but I tried to focus on highlighting the experiences that demonstrated the qualities I felt my target medical schools were looking for.

'I had decided that if my results were strong enough that I'd apply to St George's, Kings College, Imperial and UCL. This meant two BMAT medical schools and two UKCAT. I was advised to sit my UKCAT as soon as possible after my A levels so booked for the end of July and threw myself into UKCAT practice. Very tedious, but I knew it was so important for me to do well so I practised using every resource I could get my hands on. My scores were so up and down from different resources that I really had no idea how I was going to do, but was delighted to attain an average score of 750, which I later found out put me in the top quartile and in a strong position with the UKCAT Med Schools.

'BMAT was in November, so results wouldn't be known until after I'd applied, so two BMAT unis were a bit of a risk, but they were my favourites and I knew Imperial would ignore my GCSEs if I achieved a good BMAT score. So, lots more work for BMAT and then the waiting began. To my absolute delight (and shock!) my first interview invitation came from UCL, quickly followed by Imperial; I couldn't have been happier. December was spent preparing for my interviews and practising with anyone who'd listen!

'My interviews were a week apart and both being traditional interviews made it easy to prepare for them together. My interview with UCL was first and went ok, but I didn't feel I'd done my best or said everything I could of so I thought I'd get rejected. The Imperial interview went really well, so I hoped I'd done what I need to get an offer. Again, I was totally shocked and delighted to receive offers from both in under a week after each interview.

'I then received interview invites from Kings and St George's, which were MMI. I was less confident in this type of interview but attended a practice session which really helped. I attended the Kings interview and had no idea how it had gone, but received an offer. I ended up pulling out of the St George's interview before I attended, as it wasn't until April, and I had offers from my top two at that point.

'Despite UCL being my first choice all along, when it came down to it I really struggled to decide between UCL and Imperial (very fortunate position to be in I know!), as I'd convinced myself I wouldn't get an offer from UCL so had convinced myself Imperial was more likely.

'Eventually I decided on UCL and am now in my first year of medical school! I'm absolutely loving it but it still feels very surreal that I'm at one of the best medical schools in the country when I think back to my D in GCSE Chemistry!'

4 | Healthy body, healthy mind
Current issues

It is obviously impossible to know about all illnesses and issues in medicine. However, being aware of some of the issues in medicine today will be of enormous benefit, particularly if you are asked, as many candidates are, to extrapolate and elucidate on 'an issue' in an interview. Showing that you have an awareness of issues on more than a passing or superficial level demonstrates intelligence, interest and enthusiasm for medicine.

This will undoubtedly stand you in good stead next to a candidate who either is very hazy or is at worst completely unaware of a major issue in medicine. The following section illustrates, albeit briefly, some of the major issues that are currently causing debate, both in medical circles and in wider society. A little bit of awareness and knowledge can go a long way to securing and leaving a positive impression on an interview panel. This section is to be read with an eye to some of the exemplar questions given in Chapter 3.

National Health Service (NHS)

> 'The NHS employs more than 1.5 million people, putting it in the top five of the world's largest workforces, together with the US Department of Defence, McDonalds, Walmart and the Chinese People's Liberation Army.'
>
> *Source: NHS Choices,*
> *www.nhs.uk/NHSEngland/thenhs/about/Pages/overview.aspx.*

The state of the NHS is a very topical issue, and one that has elicited a lot of negative comments from practitioners. It is a very common area of questioning by interview teams.

The National Health Service was set up in 1948 to provide healthcare free of charge at the point of delivery. Accident and emergency services had been developed and had coped well with the demands of a population under bombardment during the Second World War. Some hospitals were ancient, wealthy, charitable institutions owning valuable assets such as property in London. These hospitals charged patients who could afford to pay and treated others without charge. Doctors often worked on the same basis. Other hospitals were owned and funded by local authorities. The system was supported by low-cost insurance schemes, which were often fully or partially funded by employers.

The problem perceived by the architects of the NHS was that poorer members of society were reluctant to seek diagnosis and treatment. By funding the system out of a national insurance scheme to which every employer and employee would contribute, the government conferred on all citizens (whether employed or not) the right to free healthcare without the stigma of charity.

The service has undergone a number of reforms since 1948, by far the most fundamental of which was introduced by the Conservative government in 1990 (although the coalition government's reforms in the previous administration arguably turned out to be even more far-reaching). It is important to understand what these reforms were, why they were thought to be necessary, and what the outcome has been.

By the late 1980s it was clear to the government that the NHS could not function in the future without a substantial increase in funding. The fundamental reason for this was an expected reduction in the taxpayer's contribution, linked to an anticipated increase in demand for healthcare. Let's see why this was so.

The 1990 reforms

The reforms brought about the following changes.

Hospital trusts

Hospitals (or groups of hospitals) were told to form themselves into NHS trusts, which would act as independent businesses but with a number of crucial (and market-diluting) differences. They were to calculate the cost of all the treatment they offered and to price it at cost to the GP purchasers. In addition, and on the assumption that there were inefficiencies within the system that needed rooting out, they were told to reduce this cost by 3% annually.

GP fundholders

GPs were encouraged to become 'fundholders'. They were to be empowered to buy hospital treatment for their patients at the best price they could find. If they could do this at a total cost lower than the fund, they could invest the surplus in their 'practice' for the benefit of their patients. (The fundholding scheme was not designed to cover the cost of acute emergency work.)

Hospitals

The effect of the reforms was dramatic and largely unpopular. Particularly unpopular was the assertion that old hospitals in areas of low population density were not economically viable and should be closed. St Bartholomew's Hospital in the City of London was an example. Suddenly there were winners and losers in a world that had considered itself removed from the pressures of commercial life.

The 1997 reforms

The government White Paper of 1997 (entitled *The New NHS: Modern, Dependable*) made a number of suggestions.

- The replacement of the internal market with 'integrated care'. This involved the formation of 500 primary care groups, each typically covering 100,000 patients – bringing together family doctors and community nurses – replacing GP fundholding, which ceased to exist in 1999, but which made a reappearance in the 2011 reforms (see pages 117–119).
- NHSnet. Every GP surgery and hospital would be connected via the internet – it would mean less waiting for prescriptions, quicker appointments and less delay in getting results of tests.
- New services for patients. Everyone with suspected cancer would be guaranteed an appointment with a specialist within two weeks.
- NHS Direct. A 24-hour nurse-led telephone advice and information service.
- Savings. £1 billion of savings from cutting paperwork would be ploughed back into patient care.

Rationing

Any suggestion of 'rationing' healthcare causes the public great concern. The issue hit the headlines in January 1999 when Frank Dobson (then Health Secretary) announced that, because of lack of funds, the use of Viagra (an anti-impotence drug) would be rationed: the NHS would provide Viagra only for cases of impotence arising from a small number of named causes. For example, a man whose impotence was caused by diabetes could be prescribed Viagra on the NHS, whereas if the cause was kidney failure, he would have to pay for the drug privately.

The publicity surrounding Viagra alerted people to other issues, in particular rationing by age and postcode prescribing.

Rationing by age

The charity Age Concern (now Age UK) commissioned a Gallup poll that, it claimed, revealed that older people were being denied healthcare and being poorly treated in both primary and secondary care. The BMA responded by arguing that people of different ages require different patterns of treatment or referral. They cited the example of the progression of cancer, which is more rapid in younger people and often needs more aggressive radiotherapy, chemotherapy or surgery.

Postcode prescribing

Until the formation of the National Institute for Clinical Excellence (NICE) (see below) in 1999, health authorities received little guidance on what drugs and treatments to prescribe. A well-publicised issue is that of infertility treatment (IVF). Whether or not treatment on the NHS is provided depends very much on which part of the country you live in. Across the country, about one in five infertile couples receive IVF treatment (although this figure is much higher in some areas). In February 2004 the government announced that the target would rise to four in five, and that the provision would be uniform across the country. While encouraging to prospective parents, there was (of course!) a downside: at that point, infertile couples who were eligible for IVF received up to three sets of treatment, giving a one in two chance of conception. Under the new arrangements, couples have only one set of treatment, reducing the chances of conception to one in four. After that, they have to pay for the treatment themselves.

More recently, changes in funding meant that primary care trusts (PCTs) denied women the full three treatments as they were cutting costs and in 2013 Lord Winston said that the emergence of new CCGs would make that situation worsen further as they try to balance the budgets for their area. According to the National Infertility Awareness Campaign and the Fertility Fairness website, a survey showed that 80% of CCGs in the UK were not complying with NICE regulations and commissioning the three IVF treatments, and there was at least one area that stopped providing IVF altogether. About 40% of the 50,000 women each year receiving IVF treatment are funded by the NHS. NICE has said that thousands of couples are subjected to 'postcode lotteries', with fewer than one in five – 18% in total – commissioning groups paying for the full number of IVF cycles. Women under 40 who have failed to get pregnant after two years should receive the full three cycles of IVF and those aged 40–42 should receive one, subject to certain criteria. In perspective, one cycle of IVF could cost between £1,300 and £6,000 to the NHS.

NICE

NICE was set up as a special health authority in April 1999. In April 2005 it merged with the Health Development Agency to become the new National Institute for Health and Clinical Excellence, which is still known as NICE. Its role is to provide the NHS with guidance on individual health technologies (for instance, drugs) and treatments. In the words of Professor Sir Michael Rawlins, chairman of NICE 1999–2013, 'NICE is about taking a look at what's available, identifying what works and helping the NHS to get more of what works into practice.' The government at the time acknowledged that there are variations in the quality of care available to different patients in different parts of the country, and it hoped that the guidance that NICE could provide would reduce these differences.

In a speech explaining the role of NICE, the chairman said that it was estimated that, on average, health professionals should be reading 19 medical and scientific articles each day if they are to keep up to date – in future, they could read the NICE bulletins instead.

However, NICE has not ended the controversies surrounding new treatments, since it makes recommendations based not only on clinical effectiveness but also on cost-effectiveness – something that is very difficult to judge.

For some specific examples, NICE has investigated the effectiveness of many treatments, including:

- Relenza
- hip replacement joints
- therapy for depression
- treatments for Crohn's disease
- IVF treatment (see above)
- drugs for hepatitis C
- surgery for colorectal cancer
- drugs for breast cancer (taxanes)
- drugs for brain cancer (temozolomides)
- identification and management of eating disorders such as anorexia nervosa
- laser treatment in eye surgery
- treatments for obesity
- coronary artery stents.

Full details of the results of these and other investigations can be found on the NICE website (www.nice.org.uk).

2004 reforms: foundation hospitals

NHS foundation trusts, to give them their proper title, were established to provide greater ownership and involvement of patients in their local hospitals. A board of governors was elected locally and had a large say in the running of the hospitals. Direct elections for the board of governors was designed to ensure that services were directed more closely at the local community. Hospitals have been allowed to apply for foundation trust status since April 2004. There are now 156 foundation trusts.

Figure 2 (on the following page) shows how the NHS used to be structured and the four main bodies. However, the January 2011 proposals would change this significantly (see below).

The 2011 reforms

The then Secretary of State for Health, Andrew Lansley, released the White Paper on health reform *Equity and Excellence: Liberating the NHS* on 12 July 2010 for implementation in 2011. This was the precursor to the Health and Social Care Act, which is now law; see section on NHS Structure in 2013 on page 121.

The main thrust of this White Paper was a shift in power that 'puts patients and their carers in charge of making decisions about their health and well-being'. The health service faced the biggest shake-up since its foundation. According to the *Financial Times*, the legislation to reform the NHS, prepared by civil servants, was to be far longer than the 1946 Act that set up the service.

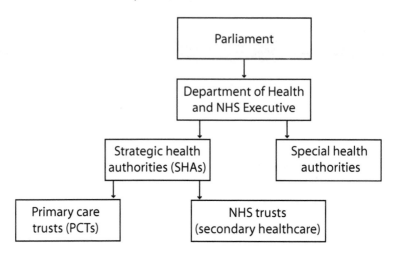

Figure 2 NHS structure pre-2011 reforms

In a statement in January 2011, Andrew Lansley outlined details of how putting 'patients and their carers in charge of making decisions' would be achieved. An £80 billion budget was to be devolved to around 500 GP consortiums who would in turn buy services such as operations or scans from hospitals and other specialists. They would have the freedom to choose who to buy the services from, including private hospitals, possibly even ones that are based outside the UK. The 151 primary care trusts would be phased out. The government predicted that this would save the NHS £5 billion, although the scheme would cost £1.4 billion to set up.

The government proposed to put the NHS in the hands of an independent panel that would control the flow of money to the GP consortiums and monitor the quality of treatment and services.

On 24 November 2011, the Department of Health published *The Operating Framework for the NHS in England 2012/13*. This was published to help the NHS move towards the system envisaged in the White Paper mentioned above. It outlined the processes required to maintain and improve the quality of the service provided over the next few years.

Not only did it refer to the standards of care required but also to the plans for financial aspects and how these could be dealt with to enable the system to run more efficiently. It stated that the four main themes proposed to enable the changes to progress were:

1. putting patients at the centre of decision making in regards to the quality of service they receive, while improving dignity and service to patients and meeting essential standards of care
2. completing the last year of transition to the new system in the NHS, building clinical commissioning groups and establishing new health and well-being boards to improve the NHS overall in the UK
3. further improve the productivity and quality of the NHS and find ways to deal with the challenges previously faced in the system, ensuring new and innovative ways of addressing the issues and updating the healthcare system
4. maintain finances, including ensuring the right to treatment within 18 weeks, which is set out in the NHS Constitution.

The previous organisation and structure

The NHS used to consist of:

- **strategic health authorities (SHAs):** in charge of planning health-care for their regions
- **primary care trusts (PCTs):** providing primary care services, such as GPs, dentists, pharmacists and district nurses
- **NHS trusts:** providing secondary care (including hospitals and ambulances)
- **special health authorities:** providing services nationally, such as NHS Blood and Transplant and NICE.

Closure of departments

In July 2012, Professor Terence Stephenson, the new chair of the Academy of Medical Royal Colleges (AoMRC), stated that many hospitals needed to close in order for there to be improvements within the NHS. He wanted ministers to downgrade NHS hospitals and ration-alise intensive care units so as not to be 'wasteful' of NHS resources. He argued that by spreading themselves too thinly, doctors are not able to give the same amount of care as they would be able to do if they were focused in one place. His arguments were designed to implement centralisation of resources.

There was also a financial reason. In September 2012, proposals were put forward to close four London A&E departments in order to plug a £332 million gap by 2014–15. The Court of Appeal has since ruled that Jeremy Hunt's announcements of cuts at Lewisham were unlawful, so not all of these closures have been implemented; however, on 30

October 2013, Hunt announced further measures to close two A&E clinics in two north-west London hospitals and replace them with 24-hour day clinics. In September 2014, Hammersmith and Central Middlesex A&E departments closed, with 22,000 patients being told to attend St Mary's Paddington. The fear was that this would affect overall performance at St Mary's. There is also a plan to demolish Charing Cross Hospital and replace it with a smaller 'local' hospital, which then would mean that all major emergency services would go elsewhere. Andy Slaughter, MP for Hammersmith, criticised these moves as 'cost-driven', with the government and the Imperial Healthcare NHS Trust needing to save a further £207 million from their budget over the next five years. In 2016, the picture once again was looking bleak as the NHS cut hospital units in response to the financial crisis. This came in response to two hospitals having to close A&E departments for children as they could no longer run them safely. Chris Hopson, chief executive of NHS Providers, went on record saying that, 'We are reaching breaking point.'

Privatisation of the NHS

In 2012, Andrew Lansley abolished the cap of 49% on private work that hospitals are allowed to do in order to secure additional funding. This opened the way for 100% privatisation of the NHS, with hospitals able to raise all of their income from private healthcare. This measure applied to all NHS services as NHS trusts were required to become self-governing by 2014. This policy put increased pressure on the coalition government, and therefore faced a struggle to go through in Parliament, as the original privatisation plans were blocked by the Liberal Democrats at the time. By September 2014 figures published showed that, instead of successful privatisation, the NHS was nearly £1 billion in debt. Therefore the next stage was devolution and the transferral of budgets to external governing bodies. In 2016, many services were being taken over by external suppliers, for example, the Virgin Care Group, which in part has a positive effect as the debt is taken on by alternative providers; at the same time though it has been lambasted in some parts as it is seen to be destabilising local hospitals as the CCG focus is on money.

Wage freezes

In 2012 approximately 70% of the NHS trusts' budgets was spent on pay. It was expected that NHS employers would ask for a pay freeze for the third year running in order to protect services. The projected savings from the pay freeze from April 2011 to March 2013 were £3.3 billion. This added to existing tensions, and trade unions warned that the NHS was losing staff over these pay conditions. A proposed 1% pay increase was halted by the government in October 2013 and with the real value of pay having consistently fallen, in 2014–15, 60% of staff did not receive a pay rise.

Changes within the NHS in 2013 and 2014

'Reforms so big they can be seen from space.'
NHS Chief Executive Sir David Nicholson

As of 1 April 2013, the structure of the NHS changed, with the legal responsibility for control of the budget being passed over to some of the new national and local services responsible for different areas of the system. This was the biggest challenge the NHS had faced since it was established in 1948.

This was the topic of intense debate over the past few years and it should be noted as well that the Health Secretary has changed since the reforms were initially planned. Jeremy Hunt took over at a time when he had to oversee the transition in power terms, with the biggest shake-up being as to who is making the decisions within the hospitals.

PCTs were replaced by Clinical Commissioning Groups (CCGs), which would be responsible for 60% of the overall NHS budget. All GPs need to belong to a CCG, and the government's idea was that GPs would be able to more effectively provide a patient's care directly, as they had the most contact with the patient. CCGs would be able to buy and plan services. Their job was to decide whether or not to pay for any care suggested by a GP for a patient, i.e. whether it is a necessity.

In most cases, care had been provided by NHS organisations; however, there were some more routine operations paid for by the NHS that were outsourced to private companies. The government introduced a new watchdog, Monitor, to ensure fair and healthy competition. Monitor is also in place to ensure that these changes do not affect overall patient care and services.

At the time, a Durham University study expressed concerns that the allocation of funding per person could widen the north–south gap, stating that the new formula being applied benefits those 'in more affluent areas'. As Lord Winston remarked, 'I suspect that by the end of 2014 we should have a really clear idea of whether this bill is thoroughly bad, or just undesirable.'

Hospital failures

In July 2013, an investigation by Sir Bruce Keogh, the medical director of the NHS, was published on instruction from David Cameron in the wake of the Stafford hospital scandal, where up to 1,200 patients died as a result of conditions. This revealed failings within 14 NHS Trusts that had the highest mortality rates over the preceding two years. The evidence showed that the depth of the problem went back to the Labour government and that it was not a result of new measures under the coalition government, but rather, of existing failures. The report showed that this could have been addressed during the previous administration and raised questions about Labour's handling of the NHS. At that time, Stafford hospital was regarded as an isolated case, with then Prime Minister Gordon Brown being assured that no similar case existed within the NHS in the United Kingdom. However, this report reveals this to have been misinformation given to the prime minister by the Healthcare Commission.

NHS spending

As the 2015 General Election was just around the corner, the NHS was inevitably a battleground for all political parties in the hope of influencing voters. The then Prime Minister and the Leader of the Opposition had several heated exchanges over the state of the NHS, not least over the topical issue of cuts and spending. The Secretary of State for Health, Jeremy Hunt, said that spending was tough but possible in a strong economy.

- Under the Labour government, the Chancellor, Alistair Darling, announced a 4% a year rise for the NHS for three years – from £90 billion in 2009 to £110 billion in 2010. The coalition government pledged to adhere to this. However, it was accused of breaking this pledge as the figure was £105.254 billion in 2012 and £95.6 billion in 2013.
- From 2010 to 2014, the NHS' spending on drugs increased by almost 50% to over £8 billion.
- Figures published in September 2014 revealed that at that point in time, the NHS was facing a debt of £1 billion.
- Much of the increase in NHS funding over this period was spent on the workforce. As a result, GP and consultant pay is now among the highest in Europe, and it is estimated that about 60% of the NHS budget is spent on staffing.
- It was reported that there are 1.7 million people working in the NHS today, and indeed the NHS employs 300,000 more staff now than it did in 1996. This has had the effect of reducing waiting lists and waiting times significantly (at least on paper).

The NHS in 2016

It is, in many ways, almost impossible to be on top of what's happening in the NHS. So, to summarise, in order to understand 2016, we need to look at the end of 2015 first. According to the published five-year plan, the NHS required an additional £8 billion by 2020, along with a restructuring of services to give greater control to GP practices. This was on top of the increase in funding of £5 billion that the government provided to the NHS within the last Parliament.

A report published by NHS England, Public Health England, the regulator Monitor, the NHS Trust Development Authority, Care Quality Commission and Health Education England set out the following figures in 2015:

- NHS England budget for 2015–16: £116.4 billion
- shortfall predicted by 2020: £30 billion
- estimated debt: £1–2 billion.

The report also highlighted the need for hospital franchises, in order to be more efficient. A hospital franchise is where a company, group or similar takes over the running of NHS services with a view to improving service (or the overseas example, where a branch of a hospital can be set up to allow funding to be channelled back to the parent site from the profits made from private patients). It is up to each area to determine which they wish to adopt from the following:

- larger GP practices can employ hospital doctors to provide extra services, including diagnostics, chemotherapy and hospital out-patient appointments
- in areas where GP services are under strain, the solution could be for hospitals to open their own surgeries
- smaller hospitals could group together to share back-office and management services
- larger hospitals could open franchises at other, smaller sites (e.g. Moorfields Eye Hospital, London)
- in order to avoid emergency admissions, hospitals could provide care directly to care homes
- volunteers could be encouraged to get more involved, with incentives such as offering council tax discounts.

Most of these options are designed to reduce the number of hospital admissions and to combat the problem of an ageing population.

The profession is sceptical and Sir Bruce Keogh has warned that patients are at risk of losing out if appropriate funding and support cannot be provided. 'There is a risk, as outlined in the report, that services may have to change or even be cut, that we will have shortages of staff, that we will have issues with waiting times and there is a risk that we will have to restrict treatments,' he said.

The NHS has been calling for more funding, otherwise it faces the real possibility of closure. The government promised it extra funding, but not immediately, calling instead for this to be front-loaded to help ease the crisis in the immediate short term. At the end of November 2015, the then Chancellor George Osborne said, 'The NHS has been heard and has been listened to', and promised a further £3.8 billion worth of funding to the NHS, effectively acquiescing to the wishes of the NHS and granting a payment largely made up front.

In 2016, the figures have been updated to reflect the following:

- anticipated rise to £133.1 billion by 2020/21, with half of that increase expected in 2016/17 and the rest to be delivered over the following years
- estimated debt: £1.8 billion.

It is worthwhile footnoting that a lot of this money will be absorbed in high and rising costs and inflation. All this is not withstanding the big news of 2016: Brexit.

Brexit

The NHS became a political battleground once again in 2016 as the Brexit vote loomed large. The Brexit campaign will be synonymous with the image of Boris Johnson on his battle bus, with the slogan, 'We send £350 million a week to the EU. Let's fund our NHS instead.' However, the slogan, like the promise, has transpired to be misleading, and the £350 million promised in Brexit has still not materialised.

So, what is the likely impact of Brexit on the NHS? Potentially, it could be seismic for the profession as a significant proportion of doctors, nurses and support staff within the NHS are EU or overseas nationals. Fast forward to Jeremy Hunt's speech at the Conservative Party conference in 2016 and his announcement that the NHS needed to be 'self-sufficient' in doctors by 2025. The solution? To train an additional 1,500 doctors. Cue uproar as the profession and medical schools scratched their heads trying to work out the feasibility of such an impractical suggestion. Given that there are over 100,000 foreign doctors that currently over 64 million people rely on, the medical schools say an extra 1,500 student doctors is going to make no difference at all.

Nevertheless, this is the modus operandi seemingly and that has a positive impact for students applying to medical school in the next few years; there has never been a better time to apply from the point of view of spaces available to you.

Weekend working

One of the most controversial issues of 2015 and 2016 was Jeremy Hunt's proposals for weekend working by doctors and consultants, which includes seven-day contracts and a cut in overtime pay. However, this is not a new issue. It has been debated for the last 20 years.

Up until now, the contract agreed by the previous Labour government has allowed consultants to opt out of non-emergency work outside of 7a.m.–7p.m. from Monday to Friday. However, Jeremy Hunt argued patients are 15% more likely to die if admitted on a Sunday than midweek. He also emphasised the fact that the salaries of 40,000 consultants have been rising since 2001. Under the new plans, therefore, there will be a new central contract that means GP practices will open, senior consultants will be on call at weekends and hospitals will now have services and clinics seven days a week, rather than five days a week.

The issue, as far as the BMA is concerned, is not a lack of support for this scheme and for an improvement in the service, but rather a lack of available resources to make this plan realistic and not stretch the NHS too thin. The government wants GP practices and hospital services available on weekends; the profession has questioned the need, saying that it needs to be funded properly.

A recent leaked memo from the NHS has shown that the profession is particularly concerned about the impact of Brexit on the seven-day services because of the possible demands and lack of resources that will be imposed on a dwindling workforce. This is among a wide array of other concerns the profession has about this plan.

NHS walkout

The walkouts started in February 2016, as tens of thousands of junior doctors went on strike over ongoing disputes regarding a change to their contracts. The BMA, which represents around 30,000 medics, said that about 76% of its members turned out to vote and of those who voted, 98% were in favour of the walkout.

Jeremy Hunt offered a 3.5% basic pay rise, at the same time as changing junior doctors' working hours; however, the BMA believed that in fact the reforms were detrimental to the safety of its members and in fact, there are some doctors who had to take a pay cut under these new guidelines. Jeremy Hunt rejected that suggestion and said instead that no doctor working within the 'legal limits of a junior doctor' would have to take a pay cut and insisted that having a maximum number of hours that they can work per week undoubtedly would improve conditions for them.

Hunt's response to the walk out by junior doctors was to state that the government would now impose the new contract on the NHS. After several walkouts, a new contract was agreed between Jeremy Hunt, the BMA and NHS Employers in May 2016. In July 2016, Mr Hunt announced that a new contract would be implemented over the course of a year, beginning from October 2016. On 3 August, 2016, the new contract came into effect, beginning in England with trainees in hospital posts and GP trainees, details of which are included in the following section.

The BMA's Junior Doctors Committee (JDC) had planned to hold three five-day walkouts between October and December 2016, but this was later called off by the BMA in September 2016, with patient safety cited as the principal concern; nonetheless, the BMA was still vocal in voicing its opposition to the introduction of the new contract. The strikes have called into question the moral grounds for abandoning sick patients to protest. What do you think the ethical implications are over walkouts? In what situations is a strike justifiable? What alternative measures can you think of instead of invoking the right to strike?

The NHS in 2017

A fair summary of the NHS would be that it has become a victim of its own success. No one can deny there are problems; however, a lot of these problems are because the NHS has got better at helping people, raising expectation and, perhaps unfairly, the service is judged on that.

In 2018, the NHS will have been running for 70 years, during which time medicine has been revolutionised with regards to innovation and care. Clinical outcomes are better, cancer survival rates are higher and the number of Care Quality Commissions (20 in total) moving out of special measures and improving is positive.

Nevertheless, pressures on the NHS are greater than ever. The last budget did not provide enough money for all of the NHS departments and Jeremy Hunt's divisive order to NHS bosses to continue with current waiting times is, within the service, considered unsustainable. The NHS itself in 2017 states that it confronts certain paradoxes.

- *'We're getting healthier, but we're using the NHS more'*. It is estimated that life expectancy has been rising by five hours a day, but alongside that the need for NHS care is more pronounced. This is largely due to the growing and ageing population, with more than half a million more people aged over 75 since 2010 and an estimated two million more in 10 years' time.
- *'The quality of NHS care is demonstrably improving, but we're becoming far more transparent about care gaps and mistakes'*. Survival rates are better but that raises public expectations.
- *'Staff numbers are up, but staff are under greater pressure'*. There are 8,000 more doctors and nurses working in the NHS since three years ago, but these staff have not been spread across all departments, rather they are clustered within certain specialisms.
- *'The public are highly satisfied with the NHS, but concerned for its future'*. Independent data from the last three decades shows that the level of satisfaction and trust from the public with the NHS is at one of its highest peaks (barring the last three years, when satisfactuion has been lower).

The NHS Five Year Forward View described three improvement opportunities: a health gap, a quality gap, and a financial sustainability gap.

Improvements made in 2017:

- action on prevention and public health
- plain packaging for cigarettes
- national diabetes prevention programme
- sugar tax agreed to reduce childhood obesity
- vaccination of over 1 million infants against meningitis and an additional 2 million children against flu
- public health campaigns including 'Be Clear on Cancer' and 'Act Fast'.

Antibiotics resistance scare

As bacteria are finding more ways of adapting and surviving antibiotics, the effectiveness of antibiotics is decreasing at a quick rate. Therefore, a campaign has been launched to urge patients to only use antibiotics when *absolutely* required; because if they use them at less critical moments, the antibiotics may not be able to counteract a more virulent illness in the future. However, it is not just the responsibility of the patient to take antibiotics as prescribed (and not save them for another illness), it is also the responsibility of doctors to appropriately prescribe them, and this is currently being addressed with doctors.

At this time, antibiotic resistance is one of the greatest threats to the safety of patients in Europe and needs careful stewardship to ensure the effectiveness of the drugs in the next decade.

Social media in medicine

It is a brave new world, and it was only a matter of time before social media and medicine found a common ground. There is an increasing trend now for the use of social networking devices in order to help patients. The latest innovation is being able to get an appointment with a GP via an app on your phone; Push Doctor and Now GP are the two leading services to do this, reportedly being able to reach over 1 million patients. This reduces waiting times and gains quicker access to doctors. Only the future will show whether this will prove as effective as seeing a GP in person.

This concept has also extended into hospitals, where a Virtual Fracture Clinic is in operation at hospitals such as the Brighton and Sussex group of hospitals in order to assess more minor injuries over the phone and then refer the patient to the virtual fracture clinic for physiotherapy exercises and monitoring, thus reducing the waiting lists of those in the hospitals waiting for appointments.

NHS's new pay and conditions

Effective from August 2016, a new contract for pay and conditions of service for doctors and dentists in national training posts have been implemented in England, with the first doctors beginning under the new terms as of October 2016. For doctors in training, the basic pay under the 2017 contract is shown in Table 6 on page 128.

The new terms and conditions for doctors (and dentists) in training in England, published 2017, are available to view on the NHS Employers website at www.nhsemployers.org/~/media/Employers/Documents/Pay%20and%20reward/FINAL%20Pay%20and%20Conditions%20Circular%20MD%2012017.pdf.

Table 6 Doctors in training

Grade	Stage of training	Grade code	Nodal point	Value(£)
Foundation Doctor Year 1	FY1	MF01	1	26,614
Foundation Doctor Year 2	FY2	MF02	2	30,805
Specialty Registrar (StR) (Core Training)	CT1	MC51	3	36,461
	CT2	MC52		
	CT3	MC53	4	46,208
Specialty Registrar (StR) (Run-Through Training) / Specialty Registrar (StR) (Higher-Training) / Specialist Registrar (SpR)	ST1/SpR1	MS01	3	36,461
	ST2/SpR2	MS02		
	ST3/SpR3	MS03	4	46,208
	ST4/SpR4	MS04		
	ST5/SpR5	MS05		
	ST6/SpR6	MS06		
	ST7/SpR7	MS07		
	ST8/SpR8	MS08		

Source: NHS Employers, www.nhsemployers.org/~/media/Employers/Documents/
Pay%20and%20reward/FINAL%20Pay%20and%2Conditions%20Circular%20
MD%2012017.pdf. Reproduced with kind permission.

In other news

Winter deaths in 2014–15 were the highest they have been since 1999, with more than 43,900 people affected. A rise in new strains of influenza was blamed; however, although this did put a strain on the NHS, it was not the cause of the rise in the number of fatalities. These were more common in women than men. This number, in fact, halved in 2015–16; however, summer deaths saw an abnormal high in 2016 in the heatwave, as the elderly, infants and those with pre-respiratory disorders were most at risk from the high temperatures. It was reported that there were 1,661 deaths on 19 July 2016 alone, when temperatures reached 33.5C, compared with a five-year average of 1,267. Climate change and global warming do have an impact on mortality at seasonal times of year. In 2017, excess winter deaths increased slightly to 34,300, though are still not close to the previous highs despite being the second highest in the past five years.

A report has also been published by a team at Imperial College London saying that babies born at the weekend are at significantly higher risk of death than if they were born midweek. In a study involving more than 1.3 million babies, deaths were 7% higher on weekends. A separate study suggested that patients who were admitted for care at weekends were at a higher risk of death within a 30-day period after leaving the hospital than those admitted on weekdays. This is something that has been well used by ministers in the ongoing argument over weekend working and the junior doctors' walkout. It has also been reported that Caesarean sections put babies at risk from becoming obese by the age of seven years or developing conditions such as asthma, as babies who are born this way lack sufficient bacteroidetes compared to babies who are born vaginally and have greater exposure to gut bacteria from the mother at birth. At the time of going to press, scientists were also warning that Caesarean sections are affecting human evolution because of a narrowing of the pelvis size, passed on through genetics in mothers who do not give birth naturally.

Hospital bed shortage made the news in December 2017; figures released by hospital trusts showed 100% bed occupancy in some cases prior to the winter bad weather. The NHS admitted that a £1 billion drive to free up 2,000 to 3,000 beds had failed to work. Even more worrying is that one in five A&E admittances require a bed and, at this moment in time, those patients face a wait on a trolley in the corridor until a bed becomes available, calling for an immediate review into how this can be rectified across the NHS as a whole.

Baby boom

In 2012, it was reported that NHS maternity wards were struggling; the Office for National Statistics reported that 729,674 babies were born, the highest number since 1972. The high birth rate continued to be a problem and was putting a strain on midwives, prompting the Royal College of Midwives to express concerns about safety, though the number of births was lower in 2013 with 695,223 live births. The College also pointed to the shortage of midwives, despite David Cameron's 2010 pledge to train 3,000 new midwives. According to the Royal College of Midwives, the NHS in England is at the moment 3,500 midwives short of being able to function effectively. In 2015–16, the number of births rose again, up 0.4% on 2014 with 697,852 births. Birth rates have risen throughout the past decade and many people say that this is a result of immigration. The media is reporting that one in six European babies are now born in the UK; however, the shortage of midwives in the future will also be attributed to our decision to leave the European Union. It is even reported that by 2026 as a result of migration, there will be a 20% rise in the number of secondary school pupils with over a half a million more students expected to start school.

Zika virus

Arguably the most topical issue of 2016, the Zika virus emanated from South America and was brought to the public consciousness through the Olympic Games when the media spotlight was firmly fixed on this continent.

First found in Uganda in 1947, the Zika virus disease is transmitted from carrier to carrier by Aedes mosquitoes, though it can also be contracted via sexual intercourse. The WHO and scientists researching the illness have concluded that the cause of the Zika virus is a combination of Guillain-Barré syndrome and microcephaly. It results in those affected having a variety of symptoms which include headaches, a mild fever, conjunctivitis, skin rash and muscle and joint pain lasting anything from two to seven days.

The complications surrounding the Zika virus are particularly dangerous for pregnant women because of the concern to birth defects in babies, resulting in abnormalities of growth and development, particularly small heads – microcephaly. In Brazil, there were 1,946 cases of Zika-related microcephaly in September 2016 when the last data was recorded.

There is no treatment for the Zika virus, though you can treat the symptoms; however, patients are encouraged to get as much rest and fluids as possible.

At this point, the Zika virus does not naturally occur in the UK. In the US, there are 5,590 cases of the Zika infection recorded. As of November 2017, no cases were confirmed in pregnant women in the UK.

Swine flu

As with the 'bird flu' scare in 2004, 2005 and 2006, the medical headlines in 2009 were dominated by the 'swine flu' (H1N1) pandemic. H1N1 was a new virus, containing genes from a number of viruses (human and animal), and so more people were affected than is normally the case for 'seasonal flu', since there is less natural immunity to a new virus.

Governments throughout the world tackled the problem in different ways – Mexico, for example, closed public buildings. Many countries embarked on a programme of vaccinations targeting the 'at-risk' groups: pregnant women, young children, and patients with respiratory and other problems.

The vaccines contain either live or dead viruses, and are administered either through injections or nasally. Antiviral drugs (zanamivir and oseltamivir) are used to treat patients who have contracted the illness.

The H1N1 pandemic raised a number of questions (some of which have been discussed in recent medical school interviews).

- Demand for the vaccine for a while outstripped supplies in many countries, which meant that governments had to decide how, and to whom, the vaccine was made available. In some countries, there was an increasingly active black market trade in the vaccine, meaning that those who could afford it and who were willing to buy it directly were able to get the vaccine, whereas poorer people could not.

- Many governments (including the UK) launched large-scale publicity campaigns soon after H1N1 was identified as being a threat, raising (some might argue) unnecessary concerns among the population, which in turn put extra pressures on already stretched health service resources. However, since then the vaccination has become part of the main flu vaccine and in 2014, the flu vaccine became available in two forms: injection and nasal defence.
- Public reaction to the condition was arguably more extreme, given that the virus was publicised as being 'swine flu' rather than H1N1 or another seasonal flu. The same had happened with 'bird flu' three years earlier.

In July 2009, the UK government's Chief Medical Officer predicted a minimum of 3,000 deaths in the UK, and mentioned an upper limit of 65,000. However, the actual number of deaths was around 500. As a result, the public has become more sceptical about warnings of pandemics. Nevertheless, flu continues to cause deaths, and in the winter of 2010–11 around 350 people in the UK had died as a result of the illness by the end of January 2011 (around 75% of the deaths were attributed to swine flu, the rest to other strains of flu). The 2011–12 flu season was the mildest on record, according to the now defunct Health Protection Agency (HPA), with a drop in the number of hospitalisations and deaths in intensive care. The H1N1 swine flu strain is one of the main viruses and is now included in the seasonal flu vaccine.

A new strain of swine flu subsequently appeared in the USA in August 2011. The strain H3N2 is different from the seasonal flu virus. There have been no cases of H3N2 in the UK or in Europe, so the risk to people over here is extremely low. In 2009, in Hong Kong, 282 people developed severe complications and 80 died from the disease. China and Hong Kong's infection rate has risen over the past few years.

In 2013, the government did a U-turn over the safety of the Pandemrix vaccine, which was given to six million people, admitting that it can cause narcolepsy, which in children can lead to learning difficulties. This, according to the Department of Work and Pensions (DWP), was likely to result in 'over 100 compensation claims', though it believed the disabilities caused by the vaccine were not severe enough to qualify for statutory compensation of £120,000. However, solicitors for those affected disagreed and said that compensation claims could be up to £1 million each. In March 2014, it was ruled in the High Court that the government should receive a bill for £60 million, with each of the 60 claimants receiving £1 million.

Swine flu returned to the UK in 2016, and was particularly prevalent among schoolchildren; however, the official guidance was that while the pandemic is over and the situation over the past few years has plateaued, it still exists in the world with evolving strains, the worst currently being in India where the numbers affected are rising. Public

Health officials have been advising parents simply on good hygiene practice to guard against an epidemic spreading. In 2017, dramatic reporting in the media of the presence of a flu strain that was only three mutations away from a strain that could kill millions has since been clarified by experts stating that the chances of three mutations actually occurring is relatively low. Nevertheless, the public are still encouraged to get winter vaccinations.

For current information, visit the WHO's Global Alert and Response pages at www.who.int/csr.

MRSA and *Clostridium difficile*

Ten years ago, most people had not heard of methicillin-resistant *Staphylococcus aureus* (MRSA). Now, horror stories abound (not all of them true) of people going into hospital to have an ingrowing toenail treated, and having to stay for six months due to picking up an MRSA infection while there. About 20–40% of people carry MRSA without even knowing it and it is harmless in most cases to healthy people. It is estimated that 100,000 people each year catch the infection in UK hospitals, and that 5,000 of them die from it. The true extent of the problem is not really known. This is not to say that there is any form of cover-up; it is simply that many people who are infected with MRSA in hospital die from causes associated with the conditions that caused them to be in hospital in the first place.

The rate of infection in the UK is one of the highest in the world because of poor hygiene in hospitals. The infection spreads via staff who handle different patients throughout the day without washing their hands in between contact with one patient and the next, or because hospital wards are not cleaned properly. If the organisms that cause MRSA get into the blood system of people weakened by illness or age, through a wound or an injection, the effects can be very serious. Since the organism is resistant to many antibiotics, it is extremely difficult to treat.

In December 2004, the *Independent* reported that the NHS was spending more than £1 billion a year in trying to prevent and treat the disease, and that over the previous seven years the number of deaths from MRSA had doubled.

In 2012, the *Guardian* published an article reporting that the number of deaths from the MRSA superbug had fallen for a fourth successive year. In 2012 figures showed that 292 people had died, compared with 364 in 2011.

In 2013, a new antibiotic was found that is proving to be effective against MRSA and anthrax. The discovery was found in an oceanic microbe and tests have been positive, according to scientists in

America. This is welcome news, as MRSA is an enormous problem. With only a sixth of NHS hospital trusts in England reporting no MRSA bloodstream infections, the government has set out a zero-tolerance policy for tackling this. More information can be found at https://improvement.nhs.uk/rresources/mrsa-guidance-post-infection-review.

One of the biggest developments in 2016 was that scientists at Imperial College London have found a way to kill food-based MRSA at source. They have found that the bacteria regulates its salt levels and is resistant to high heat levels, and so are looking into creating a treatment for other MRSA strains based on this information. In October 2016, MRSA was back in the news when six babies contracted the MRSA superbug in Rosie Hospital, Cambridge, once more bringing into question the cleanliness of hospitals. At the same time, MRSA was found in pork that had been imported from Denmark and was being sold in Asda and Tesco supermarkets, which has meant that the movement of animals is being more tightly regulated.

In 2017, public information showed that MRSA is now prevalent in the UK community and not restricted to hospitals, meaning it is harder to control the spread. After more recent cases of MRSA in private hospitals in non-surgical wards, the government has also been pressurised into tighter checks in hospital departments to ensure hygiene standards are at a satisfactory level. A total of 823 cases were reported from 2016 to 2017, which is the same as the previous year. In 2017, the general statistics were that two in 100,000 people are likely to get MRSA, though the rate is higher in the elderly: roughly 24 in 100,000 elderly males and eight in 100,000 elderly females are likely to contract the infection.

There were around 2,500 deaths attributed to *Clostridium difficile* (*C. difficile*), another hospital-acquired infection, reported in 2008, a 29% decrease from 2007. In August 2013, there were 1,646 reported deaths in 2012, 407 fewer than in 2011. Deaths had fallen for the fifth year, with the mortality rate higher among the elderly, around 0.8% when reviewed over a million cases.

In 2016, the number of *C. difficile* cases continued to decline, although it slowed due to factors affecting infection from outside the control of the NHS. CCGs have been urged to safeguard new *C. difficile* infection (CDI) objectives by placing sanctions and measures in place where breaches occur within hospitals, i.e. to ensure that good practice is always carried out. This has translated to a further decline in 2017, from 12,840 cases, indicative of a 9.2% decrease from the previous years.

Despite this, it is obviously a real problem for doctors and the medical profession as a whole. Because of this it is often a point of discussion at interview. The following questions have been asked to candidates over the last few years.

- Why are there not accurate figures about the numbers of deaths caused by MRSA and *C. difficile*?
- What is being done to try to prevent infections?
- Why might the organisms be resistant to antibiotics?
- Why are death rates now falling?

In November 2011 another report in the *Independent* stated that medical experts are warning that the world is being forced into an 'unthinkable scenario of untreatable infections'. A species of bacteria called *Klebsiella pneumoniae* (*K. pneumoniae*), known to cause urinary and respiratory diseases, has been shown to be responsible for up to 50% of blood poisoning cases in some European countries. This is particularly worrying, as over the last few years this bacteria has become more and more resistant to antibiotics, even to a group of drugs called carbapenems. These are often used as the last line of defence against multiple antibiotic-resistant bacteria.

In the UK, more than 70 patients have been found to have bacteria living in their intestines containing a gene called NBM-1. This gene causes the production of an enzyme that breaks down carbapenems and renders the antibiotic useless. If this type of bacteria spreads, which is probable without effective drugs, this will be problematic and costly for the NHS. In 2011 the UK HPA warned doctors that the drugs commonly used to treat gonorrhoea were no longer effective and that a combination of drugs should be used. Without combined drug therapy, there is a possibility that a disease as common as gonorrhoea will be untreatable in the near future. From April 2017, the government increased surveillance on this to try and reduce the number of active cases by 50% by 2021.

This is the sort of information you should be aware of when preparing yourself for interview.

Cervical cancer

Cancer of the cervix is a relatively rare type of cancer. However, it is the second most common cancer in women aged under 35, after breast cancer. In the UK, around 3,000 women are diagnosed with it each year and it is responsible for killing just under 1,000 women each year. This was brought to our consciousness by the death of Jade Goody, a Big Brother celebrity, in 2009. In the last 40 years, cervical cancer survival in the UK has increased from 46% to 63%.

The symptoms of cervical cancer are not always obvious. It may not cause any symptoms at all until it has reached an advanced stage. If cervical cancer causes symptoms, the most common is abnormal vaginal bleeding, such as between periods or after sexual intercourse.

The cervix is the lower part (or neck) of the womb. It is made of muscle tissue and is the entrance to the womb from the vagina, and it can be affected by two main types of cervical cancer.

1. Squamous cell carcinoma is the most common type of cervical cancer. It develops from the squamous cells, which are the flat cells in the outer layer of the cervix at the top of the vagina.
2. Adenocarcinoma develops from the cells that line the glands in the cervix. Adenocarcinoma can be more difficult to detect using cervical screening tests.

Cause

This type of cancer (as well as some throat cancers, due to the practice of unsafe oral sex) is caused by HPV, which stands for human papilloma viruses. Genital HPV is usually spread through intimate, skin-to-skin contact during sex and affects the skin and the moist membranes that line parts of the body, including:

- the cervix
- the anus
- the lining of the mouth and throat.

In September 2008, the NHS launched a vaccination programme for HPV. The Gardasil vaccine provides protection against the two types of HPV most responsible for the presence of cervical cancer, HPV 16 and HPV 18. In 2013, the HPV vaccination was being more widely used in England. The predictions are that it might cut cervical cancers by one third. The administering of HPV vaccine has begun in secondary schools, with girls receiving two vaccinations between six and 24 months apart, in the hope that it could save 4,500 lives a year in the future. So far it has proved positive and now there is discussion ongoing about extending the HPV vaccine to boys as well.

The prognosis is good if the cancer is caught early: early-stage cancer that is confined to the cervix can usually be successfully treated through surgery and/or radiotherapy. Also, cervical cancer can be prevented from developing if it is detected in the early stages via cervical screening, but in 2012 it was reported that one in five women are still missing their cervical cancer screenings. As reported by Cancer Research UK, women in deprived areas are at higher risk of both developing and dying from cervical cancer. One of the biggest problems that the NHS faces at the moment is that women over a certain age do not go to be screened because the process is invasive, meaning that perceptions need to be changed first in order to continue to win the fight against cervical cancer. However, if the cancer has spread to the surrounding areas, such as the vagina, bladder or lymph nodes, the outlook is less positive.

In 2016, doctors started screening women with a viral DNA test which they think is more accurate as it looks for signs of infection from the virus that causes cervical cancer. Findings published suggest that two thirds of cancer deaths had been prevented by screening, although the frequency of testing is reduced to between five to 10 years if a woman has tested negative to the presence of the cancer in the screening.

For more information visit www.cancerresearchuk.org/cancer-help/type/ cervical-cancer and www.macmillan.org.uk/information-and-support/ cervical-cancer/understanding-cancer.

Obesity

Obesity is an increasing problem throughout the UK, especially in the younger generation. With the UK at the top of the European obesity league, it is a big issue and very much an interview question. The last recorded Health Survey for England of 2015 (published in 2016) revealed that 27% of adults are clinically obese and 41% of men and 31% of women are overweight. The proportion of adults that are clinically obese has increased by 12% since 1993. The government has predicted that if measures are not taken soon, by the year 2050, 60% of the men in Britain will be obese, 50% of women and 25% of children. Obesity is defined as having a body mass index (BMI) of above 30. The annual cost is roughly £6–8 billion to the NHS (estimated to be £9.7 billion by 2050), and £49.9 billion to the wider economy.

The main causes of obesity are a combination of a lack of exercise and the consumption of excessive calories. Obesity has detrimental effects on many components of the human body, especially in later life. The extra body weight means the heart has to work harder and therefore there is an increase in blood pressure: this can lead to coronary heart disease. Atherosclerosis often occurs, which is a build-up of cholesterol and fatty substances in the lining of the arteries. This reduces the flow of blood and therefore oxygen to the heart muscle or other tissues such as the brain. Without oxygen even for a short time, cells in these tissues die. Obesity has also been shown, among other conditions, to cause respiratory problems, type 2 diabetes, and osteoarthritis due to the extra strain on the joints. The government produced a White Paper called *Healthy Lives, Healthy People: Our strategy for public health in England*. This paper, along with a document produced by the Department of Health, sets out how the problem of obesity will be dealt with over the coming years. Visit www.gov.uk/government/uploads/system/ uploads/attachment_data/file/216096/dh_127424.pdf for more details.

Childhood obesity

There has been a four-fold increase in childhood obesity in recent years; in August 2013 the media was reporting that 30% of children in the UK are obese. It is a fact that children with obese parents are 12 times more likely to be obese than children with healthier parents. However, these figures are stabilising as the NHS attempts to get on top of the problem, with initiatives such as 'Healthy lunch boxes'. The statistics are compelling though, the most shocking being that a quarter of children aged 2 to 15 years spend at least six hours every weekend day being inactive. This is the highest rate in Western Europe and contributes to the estimated overall annual cost of obesity of £6–8 billion to the NHS in the UK. For the second year in a row, the number of obese children starting primary school has increased by 0.3%, with the majority from deprived backgrounds. In order to address the dangers that obesity can have for children's health, the Chartered Society of Physiotherapy has published extensive guidelines designed to try and engage parents and young children with the idea of regular exercise in a healthy lifestyle. In light of these statistics it is clear that this issue is immensely important in terms of both preventing our children from becoming obese as well as protecting future generations.

Prior to your interview it would be worthwhile researching the sugar tax in order to see the ways the government have approached tackling childhood obesity.

Smoking

This is a section that could be quite voluminous with the amount of data available. Therefore, it is better to summarise the facts.

- Smoking is the primary cause of preventable illness in the UK.
- Smokers under the age of 40 are five times more likely to suffer a heart attack than non-smokers.
- 80% of deaths from lung cancer are caused by smoking.
- Around 80% of deaths from bronchitis and emphysema and 14% of deaths from heart disease are attributed to smoking.
- More than a quarter of all cancer deaths can be attributed to smoking.

That said, fewer than one in five persons in the UK now smoke and the smoking rate has halved since 1974 when roughly half of all men and 40% of all women smoked. This reduction is largely due to a number of measures taken to combat smoking in the past couple of decades. The most important being the ban on smoking inside public buildings, as a lot of people were suffering from second-hand smoke. In more recent years, the marketing on cigarette packaging has changed to include no branding other than a health warning. There has also been a rise in 'vaping' as an alternative to smoking.

More needs to be done though as, while the adult smoking rate is declining, other reports claim that two thirds of smokers have smoked before they are 18, which represents a significant future health warning.

What are your views on smoking and the rise of the 'vape'? Opinions should be balanced and acknowledge the preferences of everyone;

don't think purely from a medical practitioner's point of view. Interestingly, could smoking ever be medicinal?

World health

In an interview you should be able to discuss possible reasons for the changes in death rates from causes such as cancer and heart problems, and for the difference in mortality rates between men and women.

A third area that may generate questions in interviews is the state of medicine and healthcare in less economically developed countries (LEDCs). The nature of diseases and causes of death in poor countries are very different from those in the West.

Therefore, an understanding of the major water-borne diseases, such as cholera, and contagious diseases such as smallpox and/or leprosy, is of value. In addition, many of these countries have the extra burden that comes with improving incomes and life expectancies: the number of lifestyle diseases, such as cancer, is on the increase.

Rich versus poor

The world population is about 7.6 billion and growing. The biggest killers are infectious diseases, such as AIDS, malaria and tuberculosis, and circulatory diseases (17.5 million per year) such as coronary heart disease and stroke. According to the latest figures, cancer kills about 8.2 million people every year.

Infectious diseases that were once thought to be under control, such as tuberculosis, cholera and yellow fever, have made a comeback. This is due, in part, to the increasing resistance of certain bacteria to antibiotics. The antibiotics that we use now are essentially modifications of drugs that have been in use for the past 30 or 40 years, and random genetic mutations allow resistant strains to multiply.

The global economic recession

Following the 2008 financial crisis in Organization for Economic Co-operation and Development (OECD) countries, the world suffered the most serious economic downturn since the 1930s. The recent recession has created health and social challenges on a global scale, as it has had a significant and detrimental effect on the ability of countries and communities to establish a good healthcare system. In addition, the impact of earlier increases in the cost of food and fuel is estimated to have tipped more than 100 million people back into poverty.

The WHO has previously voiced its concern over certain countries that face particular risks, including those that have high debts and whose potential spending is affected by loan repayments, islands that may be affected by rising sea levels due to global warming and countries that are (or have recently been) involved in conflicts with their neighbours.

Earlier economic crises in the 1980s and 1990s started in developing countries, and a lack of focus on repairing the economies could result in more future pandemics. The global community has to spend to ensure that this does not occur. The long-term cost of inaction, especially on the part of the wealthy nations, could prove to be disastrous.

At present, the average life expectancy in OECD countries is rising, but with that so are chronic diseases such as type 2 diabetes and dementia. As most OECD countries move towards lower spending through the administration of generic medicines and shorter hospital stays to keep costs down, we are seeing an adverse effect on the population.

Infectious diseases

In the industrialised world, infectious diseases are well under control. The main threats to health are circulatory diseases (such as heart disease and stroke), cancer, respiratory ailments and musculoskeletal conditions (rheumatic diseases and osteoporosis). All of these are diseases that tend to affect older people and, as life expectancy is increasing, they will become more prevalent in the future. Many are nutrition related, where an unhealthy diet rich in saturated fats and processed foods leads to poor health.

In poorer countries, infectious diseases such as malaria, cholera, tuberculosis, hepatitis and HIV/AIDS are much more common. Malaria affects up to 212 million people a year and killed about 429,000 in 2015, and 1.7 million died from tuberculosis in 2016. According to the WHO, by the end of 2015, 36.7 million people in the world were living with HIV, with only 50% aware they have it.

Infectious diseases go hand in hand with poverty: overcrowding, lack of clean water and poor sanitation all encourage the spread of disease, and lack of money reduces access to drugs and treatment. The WHO estimates that nearly 2 million deaths worldwide each year are attributable to unsafe water and poor sanitation and hygiene.

In the WHO's 2016 update on infectious diseases, antimicrobial resistance is now threatening 'the effective prevention and treatment' of parasitic, bacterial, viral and fungal infections. It highlights this as a threat to all countries and one governments should be striving to ensure does not develop out of hand. Although antimicrobial resistance is a natural phenomenon, the result of genetic mutation and 'survival of the fittest', the effect has been amplified in recent years by the misuse of antimicrobials. Many treatments that were effective 10 years ago are no longer so, and it is a sobering thought that there have been no major new developments in antimicrobial drugs for 30 years. Given that new drugs take at least 10 years to develop and test, it is easy to see that a problem is looming. The WHO's former director-general, Dr Gro Harlem Brundtland, was quoted in the health pages of the CNN website (www.edition.cnn.com/HEALTH) as saying: 'We currently have effective medicines to cure almost every infectious disease, but we risk losing these valuable drugs and our opportunity to control infectious diseases.'

Although it is commonly stated that the overuse of antimicrobials is the cause of the problem, it might be argued that it is actually their underuse that has done the damage, since it is the pathogens that survive that cause the resistance.

Tourism also plays a part in the spread of diseases. The number of cases of malaria, yellow fever and other infectious diseases in developed countries is increasing as tourists catch the infections prior to returning to their own countries.

The effects of an ageing population

Life expectancy continues to rise (except in many sub-Saharan African countries, which have been ravaged by HIV/AIDS) because of improvements in sanitation and medical care. According to the WHO, the number of people aged 60 or over will nearly double by 2050, from about 12% of the world's population to 22%. By 2020 it is expected that the number of adults over 60 will outnumber children under the age of five. Birth rates in most countries are falling, and the combination of the two brings considerable problems. The relative number of people who succumb to chronic illness (such as cancer, diabetes or diseases of the circulatory system) is increasing, and this puts greater strain on countries' healthcare systems.

A useful indicator is the dependency ratio – the percentage of the population that is economically dependent on the active age group. It is calculated as the sum of 0- to 14-year-olds and over-65s divided by the number of people aged between 15 and 59. This ratio is rising steadily. The WHO website contains data for each country (www.who.int).

That said, there is a new baby boom in the UK, and that is introducing new strains of its own on the healthcare system (see page 129).

Life expectancy

It is a well-reported fact that the population of the UK is ageing. The ONS reports that by 2035, a projected 23% of the population will be aged over 65 years, compared to 17% when the last audit was taken in 2010.

Life expectancy figures for selected countries are shown in Table 7 (page 141). These figures could be the source of many interview questions, such as the ones listed below.

Information taken from the World Health Organization.

- Why does Japan have the highest life expectancy?
- Why does France have a higher life expectancy than the UK?
- Why are most of the countries with the lowest HALE figures located in the middle and southern parts of Africa?

You can probably guess the answers to these, but, if not, further data is available at www.who.int/gho/en.

Table 7 Life expectancy figures for selected countries

Country	Life expectancy (years)
Japan	85.26
France	81.77
UK	80.77
USA	79.13
Russia	67.72
Zimbabwe	58.56
Lesotho	53.04
Gabon	52.11
South Africa	50.3

Based on data Life expectancy at birth (years), 2017
(www.geoba.se/population.php?pc=world&type=015&year=2017&st=rank&asde=&
page=3).

HIV/AIDS

To date, some 70 million people have become infected since the disease was first recognised in 1981, and 35 million have died, according to the WHO. US actor Charlie Sheen brought the disease back into the public consciousness after announcing in 2015 that he is living with HIV. What that has done is to prompt questions about whether we are now winning against HIV/AIDS.

Table 8 (page 143) shows regional statistics for HIV and AIDS for 2016. These statistics on the world epidemic of AIDS and HIV were published by UNAIDS in 2016. Table 10 (see page 144) shows the WHO's global summary of the AIDS epidemic for 2016 published in 2017.

The WHO's current estimate of about 36.7 million people living with HIV replaces the 2006 estimate of nearly 40 million; in 2013 the WHO adopted improved information-collecting and surveillance methods. It is estimated that only one in 10 of the people who are infected with HIV or AIDS is aware of the fact. In regions where antiretroviral (ARV) therapy is freely available, there is a significant increase in the number of people who are prepared to undergo HIV/AIDS testing. This has the effect of raising awareness, which in turn reduces the stigma and encourages people to discuss and to confront the disease. This is an important factor in reducing the rate of infection. In the latest statistics, the number of newly infected people with HIV has generally continued to decline since 2001, dropping by 50% or more in 26 countries for adults and adolescents and 52% in children. It has plateaued slightly in adults, though incidents in children have continued to fall. The number of AIDS-related deaths has also declined by over 30% since its peak in 2005 and continues to drop. As you can see, the global picture shows an improvement in terms of a decrease in the number of deaths, and by and large a reduced number of new cases are being reported, but the situation is not in reverse yet. This shows a stabilisation of the global picture since last year and even signs of a further decrease in the number of people affected. In the timeframe between 2000 and 2017, the number of new HIV infections fell by 35% and the number of AIDS-related deaths fell by 28%.

It is clear that the only effective way of tackling HIV/AIDS is to adopt sustained and comprehensive programmes in affected areas; short-term measures or individual charities working in isolation have little chance of making a significant impact. The WHO has identified some of the elements that are important in an AIDS/HIV programme as:

- availability of cheap (or free) male and female condoms
- availability of free ARV therapy
- availability of effective and free treatment of all sexually transmitted diseases
- education programmes
- clear policies on human rights and effective antidiscrimination legislation
- willingness on the part of national governments to take the lead in the programme.

More than 30 vaccines have undergone trial since 1987, according to the WHO.

In 2013, researchers led by King's College London discovered a new gene that may have the ability to prevent HIV from spreading once it has entered the body. It was hoped that this would provide a way forward in creating less toxic treatments against the disease.

In the US, a recent vaccination of monkeys with Simian Immunodeficiency Virus (SIV), a much deadlier strain than HIV, proved effective in nine out of the 16 monkeys. The vaccination is based on an adapted version of the Cytomegalovirus (CMV). It is now hoped that human trials can begin; however, researchers have to make sure the vaccines are completely safe first.

In late 2016, the hope for a full cure to HIV has been raised dramatically by clinical trials carried out by scientists from five of the country's

| Region | People living with HIV 2016 (total) | New HIV infections 2016 | | | AIDs related deaths (total) 2016 | Number accessing antiretroviral therapy 2016 (total) | Number accessing antiretroviral therapy 2017 (total) |
		total	aged 15+	aged 0–14			
Eastern and southern Africa	19.4 million [17.8 million–21.2 million]	790,000 [710,000–870,000]	710,000 [630,000–790,000]	77,000 [52,000–110,000]	420,000 [350,000–510,000]	11.7 million [10.3 million–12.1 million]	12.5 million [11.0 million–13.0 million]
Asia and the Pacific	5.1 million [3.9 million– 7.2 million]	270,000 [190,000–370,000]	250,000 [190,000–370,000]	15,000 [7,700–26,000]	170,000 [130,000–220,000]	2.4 million [2.1 million–2.5 million]	2.5 million [2.2 million–2.6 million]
Western and Central Africa	6.1 million [4.9 million– 7.6 million]	370,000 [270,000–490,000]	310,000 [220,000–410,000]	60,000 [35,000–89,000]	310,000 [220,000–400,000]	2.1 million [1.9 million–2.2 million]	2.3 million [2.0 million–2.4 million]
Latin America	1.8 million [1.4 million– 2.1 million]	97,000 [79,000–120,000]	96,000 [78,000–120,000]	1,800 [1,300–2,100]	36,000 [28,000–45,000]	1.0 million [896,000–1.059,000]	1.1 million [937,000–1.1 million]
The Caribbean	310,000 [280,000–350,000]	18,000 [15,000–22,000]	17,000 [14,000–21,000]	<1,000 [<1,000–1,000]	9,400 [7,300–12,000]	162,000 [143,000–169,000]	170,000 [150,000–177,000]
Middle East and North Africa	230,000 [160,000–380,000]	18,000 [11,000–39,000]	17,000 [10,000–36,000]	1,400 [<1,000–3,300]	11,000 [7,700–14,000]	54,400 [47,800–56,500]	58,400 [51,400–60,700]
Eastern Europe and Central Asia	1.6 million [1.4 million– 1.7 million]	190,000 [160,000–220,000]	190,000 [160,000–220,000]	—*	40,000 [32,000–49,000]	434,000 [382,000–452,000]	474,000 [417,000–493,000]
Western and Central Europe and North America	2.1 million [2.0 million– 2.3 million]	73,000 [68,000–78,000]	72,000 [67,000–78,000]	—*	18,000 [15,000–20,000]	1.7 million [1.5 million–1.7 million]	1.7 million [1.5 million–1.8 million]

*Estimates were unavailable at time of publication.

Taken from UNAIDS Fact Sheet 2017. Reproduced with kind permission from UNAIDS.
Source: www.unaids.org/sites/default/files/media_asset/UNAIDS_FactSheet_en.pdf.

Table 9 Regional statistics for HIV and AIDS for 2015

Region	People living with HIV 2015	New HIV infections 2015		AIDS-related deaths 2015 (total)
	total	total	children	
Eastern and southern Africa	19.0 million	960,000	56,000	470,000
Latin America and the Caribbean	2.0 million	100,000	2,100	50,000
Western and Central Africa	6.5 million	410,000	66,000	330,000
Asia and the Pacific	5.1 million	300,000	19,000	180,000
Eastern Europe and Central Asia	1.5 million	190,000	-	47,000
Middle East and North Africa	230,000	21,000	2,100	12,000
Western and Central Europe and North America	2.4 million	91,000	-	22,000
Global	36.7 million	2.1 million	145,200	1.1 million

Taken from UNAIDS Fact Sheet November 2016.
Reproduced with kind permission from UNAIDS.

Table 10 Global summary of the AIDS epidemic for 2017 (published 2017)

	Total (in millions)	Adults (in millions)	Children (under 15 years old) (in millions)
Number of people living with HIV	36.7	34.9	2.1
People newly infected with HIV in 2016	1.8	1.9	0.16
AIDS deaths in 2016	1.0	1.0	0.11

Based on data Global summary of the AIDS epidemic.
Reproduced with kind permission from UNAIDS. Source: www.unaids.org/sites/
default/files/media_asset/UNAIDS_FactSheet_en.pdf.

leading universities. They found that in trials on a 44-year-old man, the virus became completely undetectable in human blood. It is still too early to say it will be a full cure; however, scientists are hopeful these positive indications will continue. In 2017, researchers have developed a molecule to 'kick and kill' HIV, which could rid some or all of the virus from people who are infected.

Women and AIDS

In some sub-Saharan African countries more than 75% of young people living with HIV/AIDS are women, and in the sub-Saharan region as a whole the rate of infection among women in the 15 to 24 age group is over three times greater than that among males in the same age group. Yet surveys in parts of Zimbabwe and South Africa indicate that nearly 70% of women have only ever had one sexual partner, and education programmes targeting women have been relatively effective. The main cause of the spread of the infection in Africa (and increasingly in India and South-East Asia) is through men having unprotected sex with sex workers and subsequently passing on the disease to their partners. This, in turn, increases the incidence of mother-to-baby infection.

Ebola

The spread of the deadly Ebola virus recently put many countries on alert. First identified in Africa in 1976, it is a rare but potentially fatal disease, currently with a 25%–90% fatality rate. As of 27 March 2016, the numbers of cases of Ebola reported since March 2014 are:

- Guinea: 3,811 cases; 2,543 deaths
- Liberia: 10,675 cases; 4,809 deaths
- Sierra Leone: 14,124 cases; 3,956 deaths
- All countries: 28,646 cases; 11,323 deaths

The WHO officially declared West Africa Ebola-free in March 2016, with the caveat that new flare-ups are likely to occur. However, this is remarkable when you consider the difficulties the area faced during this crisis (see numbers above). What it shows is that the medical profession appears to have found a way to contain it in developing countries. The most recent case in 2017 was in the Democratic Republic of Congo. The outbreak has now been declared to be at an end by the WHO.

There are five known species of the Ebola virus. They cause Ebola Virus Disease (EVD), previously known as Ebola Haemorrhagic Fever. The first cases of the disease occurred in 1976 and appeared simultaneously in the Democratic Republic of Congo (near the Ebola river, hence the name) and in Sudan. The outbreak in West Africa in March 2014 was the most severe since then, accounting for the lives of over 11,000 people.

The symptoms are very similar to other diseases common to that part of the world, such as typhoid fever, malaria and meningitis, making diagnosis potentially very difficult. Fever, muscle pain, headache, sore throat, vomiting, diarrhoea, rash and internal and external bleeding are all likely. The symptoms may take 21 days to develop from initial exposure to the virus, and the person is infectious only after the onset of the symptoms.

The natural host for the Ebola virus is a particular species of fruit bat, and contact with the body fluids and tissues from these animals or others such as infected primates can often be the initial source of infection. Most transmission in humans is caused by person-to-person contact and again via body-fluid exchange. It is a common way of health workers becoming infected. It is vital that health workers take effective precautions so as not to come into contact with these fluids. During the outbreak's peak, many airlines took the precaution of reducing the number of flights to and from countries that had reported recent cases of the virus, with airports also screening passengers upon landing. These entry and travel restrictions have mostly all been lifted now under growing pressure from the UN; however, there are restrictions in place in some countries that are not yet Ebola-free.

There is no totally effective treatment for Ebola yet. The main plan involves primarily intravenous and oral rehydration with clean water and minerals and salts. The very latest research in drug development is based on using the serum antibodies from sufferers who have survived the disease. A WHO-led trial for a new vaccine for Ebola has started to prove highly protective against the virus, according to results of the testing on 11,841 people in Guinea in 2015. No signs of the virus in these cases ever occurred and, in 2017, it was considered that there was a vaccination against the disease that could be manufactured and give high positive results.

Natural disasters

In the past couple of years, events such as the earthquake in Nepal, Super Typhoon Haima in the Philippines and Hurricane Matthew which hit Haiti have tended to focus the world's attention on the devastation caused by a natural disaster, particularly if it happens in the less developed world. There are new examples that you could include every year. However, don't forget that developed nations are also affected – for example, the severe earthquakes in Italy and New Zealand in 2016, the devastation on the east coast of America after Superstorm Sandy in 2012, the tornado in Moore, Oklahoma in 2013, and the emergence of Thunderstorm Asthma in Australia which is proving a danger to people.

Whenever a natural disaster occurs (floods, earthquakes or other events that displace people from their homes), food supplies are affected and clean water supplies are contaminated, which results in an enormous increase in infectious diseases such as diarrhoea, cholera and typhoid. In addition, malnutrition and difficulties in providing adequate medical treatment contribute to the number of deaths. Obviously, Western nations can cope with these emergencies much better than poor ones.

The earthquake in Pakistan in October 2005 killed 73,000 people, left another 70,000 injured and made 3 million homeless. As well as the problems associated with a lack of clean drinking water, it is estimated that in the three months following the earthquake, 13,000 women delivered babies and many of these mothers and their children needed immediate medical attention. In April 2015 an earthquake in Nepal killed over 9,000 people and injured more than 23,000. It also triggered the worst-ever avalanche on Mount Everest, resulting in the loss of 19 lives.

Even the world's richest and most powerful country, the US, was unable to cope with the aftermath of Hurricane Katrina, which hit the Gulf of Mexico in August 2005 and killed over 1,300 people, leaving a further 375,000 homeless. Superstorm Sandy killed 110 people and left thousands more homeless, with $50 billion worth of damage caused across the affected areas of the US. The tornado in Moore killed 25 people, injured 377, destroyed 1,150 homes and caused $2 billion of damage; and Hurricane Matthew killed 49 people in the US and caused $10.5 billion worth of damage, making it the tenth costliest in history. In 2017, hurricanes Harvey, Irma and Maria changed the face of the Caribbean and affected millions of people. Some communities' infrastructure were wiped out, leaving them facing long-term health effects through the spread of disease as a result of poor living conditions. Disasters with human causes, particularly wars and persecution of ethnic groups – the current migration crisis from Syria and the Middle East to western Europe is a prime example of this – also cause people to be displaced from their homes, and many of the same problems caused by natural disasters are prevalent.

Moral and ethical issues

Lastly, the weighted and complex questions that have a moral and/or ethical dimension constitute a very relevant and current area that has caused large amounts of discussion – and, indeed, can often polarise opinion. Many medical students with whom we have spoken tell us that, almost without exception, either one or several of the following issues were discussed at the interview stage.

Genes: medical and ethical issues

Many illnesses are thought to be caused by defective genes: examples are cancer, cystic fibrosis and Alzheimer's disease. The defects may be hereditary or can be triggered by external factors such as ionising or solar radiation. The much-hyped dream of medical researchers, especially in the US, is that the affected chromosomes could be repaired, allowing the body to heal itself.

To make this dream come true, scientists need to discover which gene is causing the problem and work out how to replace it with a healthy one. Great progress has been made in solving the first part of the puzzle, thanks to a gigantic international research project known as the Human Genome Project, which has as its aim the identification of every human gene and an understanding of what effect it has. The full sequence was published in early 2000. Many links have been made between diseases and specific genes, but the techniques for replacing the defective genes have yet to prove themselves effective.

Two methods have been proposed.

1. The healthy gene is incorporated into a retrovirus which, by its nature, splices its genetic material into the chromosomes of the host cell. The virus must first be treated in order to prevent it causing problems of its own. This 'denaturing' reduces the positive effects and, to date, the trials have been unconvincing.
2. The healthy gene is incorporated into a fatty droplet, which is sprayed into the nose in order to reach cells in the lining of the nose, air passages and lungs, or injected into the blood. It was hoped that this method would be effective against the single defective gene that causes cystic fibrosis but, again, the trials have yet to prove successful.

To make matters more complicated, it turns out that many of the illnesses that are genetic in origin are caused by defects in a wide number of genes, so the hoped-for magic bullet needs to be replaced by a magic cluster bomb – and that sounds suspiciously like the approach used by conventional pharmaceuticals. Since 1990, when gene therapy for humans began, about 300 clinical trials (involving diseases ranging from cystic fibrosis and heart disease to brain tumours) have been carried out, with very limited success.

At the forefront of today's exploration in the field, the National Human Genome Research Institute is continuing to make progress with mapping the human genome, looking at how variations in genes affect a disease. At the moment, they are continuing to research and explore the links between environment and genetics to aid the prevention and treatment of illnesses such as asthma and arthritis.

Genetic engineering

Genetic engineering is the name given to the manipulation of genes. There is a subtle difference between genetic engineering and gene therapy: specifically, that genetic engineering implies modification of the genes involved in reproduction. These modifications will then be carried over into future generations.

One of the reasons for considering these ideas is to try to produce enhanced performance in animals and plants. The possibility of applying genetic engineering to humans poses major ethical problems and, at present, experiments involving reproductive cells are prohibited. Nevertheless, one form of genetic engineering known as genetic screening is allowed. In this technique, an egg is fertilised in a test tube. When the embryo is two days old, one cell is removed and the chromosomes are tested to establish the sex and presence of gene defects. In the light of the tests, the parents decide whether or not to implant the embryo into the mother's womb.

Taken to its logical conclusion, this is the recipe for creating a breed of supermen. The superman concept may be morally acceptable when applied to racehorses, but should it be applied to merchant bankers?

How would we feel if a small, undemocratic state decided to apply this strategy to its entire population in order to obtain an economic advantage? Could we afford to ignore this challenge?

The fundamental argument against any policy that reduces variation in the human gene pool is that it is intrinsically dangerous because, in principle, it restricts the species' ability to adapt to new environmental challenges. Inability to adapt to an extreme challenge could lead to the extinction of our species.

Since 2012, the Nobel prize-winning discovery of re-programming cells has offered scientists a way around the ethical issues of human embryos. Stem cells can be implanted with the source codes required to re-programme other cells within the body, acting as a control centre. This is still relatively new and presents safety as well as ethical concerns.

In 2016, scientists made an important discovery in the field of immune engineering, which is helping to make a breakthrough in cancer treatment. They have managed to engineer T-cell receptors (which are essential to the immune system) to attack specific cancer antigens. This has the potential to make major advances in the fight against cancer in the future and is currently being extensively researched.

Also, the President of the Royal Society, Sir Venki Ramakrishnan, has asked for the debate into the genetic engineering of human beings to be reopened, in order to help those who are genetically expected to inherit serious diseases. However, this is a debate that reaches far beyond the world of science, and the argument over ethics has once again been brought to the fore. The stand-off is up to each individual to decide whether the debate is standing in the way of progress or whether it is right to stop ourselves before we take technology ultimately too far.

Euthanasia and assisted deaths

Euthanasia is illegal in the UK, and doctors who are alleged to have given a patient a lethal dose of a medication with the intention of ending that person's life will be charged with manslaughter or murder, depending on the circumstances surrounding each case. UK law also prohibits assisting with suicide. The Suicide Act of 1961 decriminalised suicide in England and Wales, but assisting a suicide is a crime under that legislation.

Section 2(1) of the Suicide Act 1961 provides:

> 'A person who aids, abets, counsels or procures the suicide of another, or an attempt by another to commit suicide, shall be liable on conviction on indictment to imprisonment for a term not exceeding 14 years.'

However, in order to prove the offence of aiding and abetting it is necessary to prove firstly that the person in question had taken their own life and, secondly, that an individual or individuals had aided and abetted the person in committing suicide.

In December 2004, a High Court judge allowed a husband to take his wife (referred to as Mrs Z in the case) to Switzerland – where the law on euthanasia is different – to help her to die. Mrs Z was unable to travel alone as she had an incurable brain disease, but the local authorities had tried to prevent her husband taking her. It was reported in the *Observer* in December 2004 that an estimated 3% of GPs in the UK had helped patients to die. The *Observer* also stated that in a poll of doctors, 54% favoured legalising euthanasia. The BMA website provides detailed information on the law in a number of countries, and the ethical considerations behind euthanasia.

The debate is ongoing, and and has been prevalent over the past decade, a prime example of which is the case of the rugby player Daniel James, who in 2007 became a tetraplegic after a rugby accident. After several attempts at suicide in the UK he was directed to Dignitas in Switzerland, where he committed suicide in 2008. The police investigated the acts of Daniel's parents and a family friend and concluded that there would be sufficient evidence to prosecute each of them for an offence of aiding and abetting Daniel's suicide. However, contrary to the law (see above), it was decided that, on the particular facts of this case, a prosecution would not be in the public interest. It was interesting that the police took this stance, but it does reflect the complexity of such ethical matters.

In another case, as reported by the BBC, in 2009 a woman with multiple sclerosis made legal history by winning her battle to have the law on assisted suicide clarified. Debbie Purdy wanted to know if her husband would be prosecuted if he helped her end her life in Switzerland. Five of the then called 'Law Lords' ruled that the Director of Public Prosecutions (DPP) must specify when a person might face prosecution. Ms Purdy said that the Law Lords' decision was 'a huge step towards a more compassionate law'.

In October 2014 the DPP published its updated policy on prosecuting assisted suicide cases. The Crown Prosecution Service website gives details of the public interest factors against prosecution. These include:

1. the victim had reached a voluntary, clear, settled and informed decision to commit suicide

2. the suspect was wholly motivated by compassion
3. the actions of the suspect, although sufficient to come within the definition of the offence, were of only minor encouragement or assistance
4. the suspect had sought to dissuade the victim from taking the course of action which resulted in his or her suicide
5. the actions of the suspect may be characterised as reluctant encouragement or assistance in the face of a determined wish on the part of the victim to commit suicide
6. the suspect reported the victim's suicide to the police and fully assisted them in their enquiries into the circumstances of the suicide or the attempt and his or her part in providing encouragement or assistance.

Source: www.cps.gov.uk/legal-guidance/policy-prosecutors-respect-cases-encouraging-or-assisting-suicide. Contains public sector information licensed under the Open Government Licence v2.0.

More recently, the Tony Nicklinson case in March 2012 brought this law into question again. Tony Nicklinson was paralysed from the neck down after a stroke, leaving him with 'locked-in syndrome'. While High Court judges sympathised with his case, they refused his appeal to grant immunity to a doctor to help him end his life, stating that it was for Parliament to decide, not the judicial process. Even though Tony Nicklinson died of pneumonia six days after this hearing, having starved himself in response to the verdict, the family continue to fight this ruling for other sufferers in similar predicaments. As reported in the previous chapter, in 2013 the Court of Appeal rejected cases from Jane Nicklinson and Paul Lamb (who was paralysed after a road accident) despite intervention from the British Humanist Association (BHA), which was seeking to lend its support. A second case was won, however, in a case for a man known only as 'Martin'. A ruling from two Court of Appeal judges said the law should be 'spelt out unambiguously' over whether those seeking to help would be prosecuted, with the DPP now forced to clarify and possibly having to state that prosecutions will not be made against those who aid this decision.

In June 2015, a Bill proposed by Lord Falconer completed its first reading in the House of Lords. If approved by both Houses of Parliament, this new law would allow terminally ill, mentally competent adults, to request that a doctor provide them with life-ending medication. The details of how this medication would be administered to a patient, particularly where they were incapable of self-administration, are yet to be confirmed but what is significant is that the doctor would no longer face criminal prosecution for taking a positive step to help end a patient's life. The current law only allows doctors to withdraw medication and sustenance from a patient in a persistent vegetative state.

In 2015, Simon Binner again brought this issue to the media as he posted details of his condition – motor neurone disease – along with the dates of his death and funeral on his LinkedIn page, before flying to Switzerland for assisted suicide; thus continuing to raise the debate about dignity over legality. Following on from Lord Falconer's bill, which simply ran out of time before the General Election, 2015 also saw the Assisted Dying Bill introduced by Rob Marris – the first real move to change UK law on the right to die – which was overwhelmingly rejected by MPs at the second reading, who did not want to change such a controversial law. It is likely that the motion will go before Parliament again in the future as it is an issue which keeps coming up.

You can find more information about the DPP's policy on assisted suicide at www.cps.gov.uk/publications/prosecution/assisted_suicide.html.

Abortion

Even recently there was new controversy regarding abortion, as the BMA issued guidance advising doctors that 'there may be circumstances in which termination of pregnancy on fetal grounds would be lawful'. As reported in the *Telegraph*, there was a backlash from MPs who have criticised the BMA for trying to redefine abortion laws. In the wake of the controversial decision of the CPS not to prosecute two doctors who were secretly filmed offering to abort selected-sex babies, the DPP warned that the guidance for doctors needs urgently to be updated. The current BMA guidance suggests that it is 'unethical' to terminate a pregnancy on the grounds of sex alone, but it also says that the wishes and situation of the mother should be considered. The Law and Ethics of Abortion BMA Views report of November 2014, says that in England, Scotland and Wales, provided the criteria from the Abortion Act 1967 are fulfilled, then abortion is lawful. It goes on to say that unless it is necessary to save the life of the mother, doctors have a right to conscientious objection should they wish.

One in three women will have an abortion before they are 45 years old, and in 2016 there were 190,406 abortions in the UK. Yet, without certain conditions being met, abortion is still illegal. Indeed, it is the subject of controversy at the moment in Northern Ireland, where there are more restrictions on abortion than there are in England, Scotland and Wales.

This is an issue to keep updated on as it is a prevalent topic within the medical profession.

The internet

The internet provides the medical world with many opportunities but also some problems. The wealth of medical information available on the internet enables doctors to gain access to new research, treatments and diagnostic methods quickly. Communication between doctors, hospitals, research groups and governing bodies is simple, and news (e.g. the outbreak of a disease) can be sent around the world in a matter of minutes. The internet can also be used to create web-based administrative systems, such as online appointment booking for patients.

For patients, the internet can be used to find out about treatments for minor illnesses or injuries without having to visit a doctor or a hospital. A good site to investigate is NHS Choices (www.nhs.uk), which also provides patients with a search engine to locate local doctors.

Not all of the information available, however, is reliable. Anyone can set up a website and make it appear to be authoritative. Type 'cancer', for example, into Google and you will find nearly 2 billion sites or articles listed! Some of these are extremely useful, such as information sites provided by doctors, health organisations or support groups. However, there are also an enormous number of sites selling medicines or treatments (which in the best cases may be harmless, but could also be extremely dangerous) and quack remedies. Even if the medication that is purchased is the correct one for the condition, the drugs could be fake, of inferior quality or the incorrect dosage. In many cases, side-effects from one type of medication need other drugs to control them.

The internet also allows patients to self-diagnose, but the dangers of this range from attributing symptoms to something life-threatening (and then buying harmful drugs from another website) to gaining reassurance that the condition is harmless when it might be something more serious.

5 | The placebo effect
Results day

The A level results will arrive at your school on the third Thursday in August. For International Baccalaureate (IB) qualifications results day will be in the first week of July and for students studying in Scotland it will be the first week of August. The medical schools will have received them a few days earlier. You must make sure that you are at home on the day the results are published. Don't wait for the school to post the results slip to you. Get the staff to tell you the news as soon as possible. If you need to act to secure a place, you may have to do so quickly. This chapter will take you through the steps you should follow – for example, you may need to use the Clearing system because you have good grades but no offer. It also explains what to do if your grades are disappointing.

What to do if things go wrong during the exams

If something happens when you are preparing for or actually taking the exams that prevents you from doing your best, you must notify both the exam board and the medical schools that have made you offers. This notification will come best from your head teacher and should include your UCAS number. Send it off at once; it is no good waiting for disappointing results and then telling everyone that you felt ghastly at the time but said nothing to anyone. Exam boards can give you special consideration if the appropriate forms are sent to them by the school, along with supporting evidence.

Your extenuating circumstances must be convincing. A 'slight sniffle' won't do! If you really are sufficiently ill to be unable to prepare for the exams or to perform effectively during them, you must consult your GP and obtain a letter describing your condition.

The other main cause of underperformance is distressing events at home. If a member of your immediate family is very seriously ill, you should explain this to your head teacher and ask him or her to write to the examiners and medical schools.

With luck, the exam board will give you the benefit of the doubt if your marks fall on a grade border. Equally, you can hope that the medical school will allow you to slip one grade below the conditional offer, although this is rare now that there are so many applicants chasing a small number of places. If things work out badly, then the fact that you declared extenuating circumstances should ensure that you are treated sympathetically when you reapply through UCAS.

The medical school admissions departments are well organised and efficient, but they are staffed by human beings. If there were extenuating circumstances that could have affected your exam performance and that were brought to their notice in June, it is a good idea to ask them to review the relevant letters shortly before the exam results are published.

What to do if you hold an offer and get the grades

If you previously received a conditional offer and your grades equal or exceed that offer, congratulations! You can relax and wait for your chosen medical school to send you joining instructions. One word of warning: you cannot assume that grades of A*AB satisfy an AAA offer. This is especially true if the B grade is in chemistry. Call your chosen university and confirm that you have met your offer.

What to do if you have good grades but no offer

Very few schools keep places open and, of those that do, most will choose to allow applicants who hold a conditional offer to slip a grade rather than dust off a reserve list of those they interviewed but didn't make an offer to. Still less are they likely to consider applicants who appear out of the blue – however high their grades. That said, in August 2016, St George's became the first UK medical school to offer places for its medicine course through Clearing, paving the way for other schools to follow suit and, indeed, Bristol and Liverpool were offering places in 2017.

If you hold three A grades but were rejected when you applied through UCAS, you need to let the medical schools know that you are out there. The best way to do this is by email. Contact details are listed in the UCAS directory. If you live nearby, you can always deliver a letter in person, talk to the office staff and hope that your application will stand out from the rest.

Set out below is sample text for an email. Don't copy it word for word!

To: Mrs Lister
Subject: Application to study medicine at Rushmere University

Dear Mrs Lister
UCAS no. 16-024680-8

I applied to study medicine at Rushmere University this year. I regrettably was rejected as a result of my interview/without an interview, which at the time I was disappointed to hear. However, I did not let it deter me but instead used it as my spur. Today I received grades:

Biology – A
Chemistry – A*
Mathematics – A*

While I appreciate this is a very busy time of year for you and that it is non-standard to take applicants at this stage of the year, I am contacting you to see if, after results day, there were any places still at Rushmere University to study medicine. I learned a great deal from my interview experience previously and I would be very willing to attend another interview at short notice to demonstrate that I have taken on board the advice I was given.

I have informed my referee of my decision to write to you and she is willing to support my application and give you any information you require. Her details are:

Rachel Gaw
tel: 0198 7654 3210
email: r.gaw@royalessexcounty.sch.uk

I look forward to hearing from you.

Yours sincerely
Charlotte Stevenson

Don't forget that your UCAS referee may be able to help you. Try to persuade him or her to ring the admissions officers on your behalf – he or she will find it easier to get through than you will. If your referee is unable or unwilling to ring, then he or she should, at least, email a note in support of your application. It is best if both emails arrive at the medical school at the same time. In order for your referee to be able to help you, you need to put his or her name on the UCAS application in the section that asks you to nominate someone who can act on your behalf.

If you are applying to a medical school that did not receive your UCAS application, ask your referee to email or fax a copy of the application. In general, it is best to persuade the medical school to invite you to arrange for the UCAS application to be sent.

If, despite your most strenuous efforts, you are unsuccessful, you need to consider applying again (see below). The other alternative is to use the Clearing system to obtain a place on a degree course related to medicine and hope to be accepted on the medical course after you graduate.

UCAS Adjustment process

The UCAS Adjustment option is for students who have accepted an offer of a place and then achieve higher grades. A typical case might be the student who accepts a CCC offer to study bioengineering and then achieves AAA. He or she then has a small period of time (usually a week) to register for Adjustment in order to be able to approach universities that require higher grades.

It is unlikely that potential medics would be able to gain places this way, since there are very few medical places available in the post-results period and those that are available would normally be allocated to students who applied for medicine in the first place. But if you are in this situation, there is nothing to be lost by contacting the medical schools to see if they can consider you. Details can be found on the UCAS website.

What to do if you hold an offer but miss the grades

If you have only narrowly missed the required grades, it is important that you and your referee contact the medical school to put your case before you are rejected. Sample text for another email follows below.

To: Mrs Lister
Subject: Application to study medicine at Rushmere University

Dear Mrs Lister
UCAS no. 16-024680-8

I have a place to study medicine at Rushmere University this year. However, I am afraid that having received my results, I found that I have missed my offer. Today I received grades:

Biology – B
Chemistry – A
Mathematics – A*

As you can see, I just missed my offer by one grade in Biology, though I received a higher grade than anticipated in Mathematics. Therefore, I was wondering if you could guide me as to whether my grades are still applicable for my place or what the next steps are if my place is to be rescinded. I worked incredibly hard for the exams; however, there were extenuating circumstances affecting

---

my exams at the time and this has influenced my Biology result. I offer this only as context in the hope that I could seek a conversation with you to explain.

I have informed my referee of my decision to write to you and she is willing to support my application and give you any information you require. Her details are:

Rachel Gaw
tel: 0198 7654 3210
email: r.gaw@royalessexcounty.sch.uk

I look forward to hearing from you and remain resolute and determined to achieve my place at Rushmere University, as for me, it is without question where I wish to develop and train as a doctor.

Yours sincerely
Charlotte Stevenson

If this is unsuccessful, you need to consider retaking your A levels and applying again (see below). The other alternative is to use the Clearing system to obtain a place on a degree course related to medicine and hope to apply to a medical course after you graduate.

Retaking A levels

The grade requirements for retake candidates are normally higher than for first-timers (usually A*AA). You should retake any subject where your first result was below B and you should aim for an A grade in any subject you do retake. It is often necessary to retake a B grade, especially in chemistry – take advice from the college that is preparing you for the retake.

AS and A level units (under the old system) in Phase One legacy subjects (i.e. biology, business studies, chemistry, economics, English literature, history, physics, psychology and sociology) can no longer be retaken, Phase Two subjects are due for final examinations in 2018. Retakes on the A level reformed syllabuses will be allowed, with examinations taking place in the summer exam session, although you will not be able to resit individual modules; you will need to retake the whole A level. If you are retaking coursework units you will need to check when this can be done with the exam board. More information on what will be available for examination in which year until 2019 can be found at www. gov.uk/government/publications/get-the-facts-gcse-and-a-level-reform/get-the-facts-as-and-a-level-reform.

The most important point to bear in mind is that, under the new reforms, should you wish to retake any A level on the new reformed syllabus, it will be a risk because, unlike the old system that took the best grade out of your original A level and your retake, this system will take the next grade, thereby effectively losing the previous grade; so, worthwhile if you have a C grade or lower and need to improve by a large margin, but if you already have a B grade you need to weigh up whether you want to risk losing that grade.

Check with your college or school on its provisions for students wanting to retake. It is also possible to retake A levels at some further education colleges. Interviews to discuss this are free and carry no obligation to enrol on a course, so it is worth taking the time to talk to their staff before you embark on A level retakes.

It is possible to resit IB examinations. This is available in either November or May, though you would have to complete within three opportunities to complete the qualification. You can retake a Scottish Higher in a separate academic year and the same is true for Advanced Highers, but not in all subjects. You would have to register again for, and then resit, the Advanced Highers. The same applies for the IB examinations, as you would effectively need to sit the whole qualification again.

Reapplying to medical school

Many medical schools discourage retake candidates (see Table 12 on pages 206–208), so the whole business of applying again needs careful thought, hard work and a bit of luck. The choice of medical schools for your UCAS application is narrower than it was the first time round. Don't apply to the medical schools that discourage retakers unless there really are special, extenuating circumstances to explain your disappointing grades. Among the excuses that will not wash are the following.

- I wasn't feeling too good on the day of the practical exam, knocked over my Bunsen and torched the answer book.
- My dog had been ill for a week before my exams and only recovered after the last paper (and I've got a vet's certificate to prove it).
- I'd spent the month before the exams condensing my notes onto small cards so that I could revise effectively. Two days before the exams, our house was broken into and the burglar trod on my notes as he climbed through the window. The police took them away for forensic examination and didn't give them back until after the last paper (and I've got a note from the CID to prove it).

Some reasons are acceptable to even the most fanatical opponents of retake candidates:

- your own illness
- the death or serious illness of a very close relative.

Consider, in addition, your age when you took the exams. Most medical schools will accept that a candidate who was well under the age of 18 on the date of sitting A levels may deserve another attempt without being branded a 'retaker'.

These are just guidelines, and the only safe method of finding out if a medical school will accept you is to ask it. Text for a typical email is set out below. Don't follow it slavishly and do take the time to write to several medical schools before you make your final choice.

To: Mrs Lister
Subject: Application to study medicine at Rushmere University

Dear Mrs Lister
UCAS no. 16-024680-8

I hope you don't mind the personal approach but I was wondering if I could ask for your advice. I am hopeful of applying to Rushmere University this year but I am retaking my A levels.

This year, I received grades
Biology – B
Chemistry – B
Spanish – B

I note that you encourage retake applicants in specific circumstances; however, I am not sure if I would be eligible and I hope that you will be able to advise me. I cannot give any extenuating circumstances but I can give assurances that I have learned valuable lessons from the examinations that I am now translating into my resit courses this year. They have become my incentive and I am even more determined for this year, a quality I think will stand me in good stead in the medical profession.

I was struck by Rushmere University when I visited because of the world class teaching, the resources, the campus and accommodation and in truth, just the whole feel of the place. It is why I am taking this step to contact you directly as I am determined to become a part of the university next year.

I have informed my referee of my decision to apply to you and she is willing to support my application and give you any information you require. Her details are:

Rachel Gaw
tel: 0198 7654 3210
email: r.gaw@royalessexcounty.sch.uk
I look forward to hearing from you.

Yours sincerely
Charlotte Stevenson

Notice that the format of your email should be:

- opening paragraph
- your exam results: set out clearly and with no omissions
- any extenuating circumstances: a brief statement
- your retake plan, including the timescale
- a request for help and advice
- closing formalities.

Make sure that it is brief, clear and well presented. Apart from the care needed in making the choice of medical school, the rest of the application procedure is as described in the first section of this book.

The same advice applies if you are reapplying with qualifications other than A levels. If you did not get a place but now have the grades required, then you can reapply, but make sure you talk to the medical schools first. If you have not got the grades, then you need to look at what routes are available. If you do not resit the IB, you will need to look at A levels or Foundation programmes in order to reach the requisite entry requirement for a medicine course. If you have taken Scottish Highers, depending on the subject, you are able to retake again in a new academic year. Either way, you must make sure that you gain the necessary qualifications in the next sitting – even though this will allow entry to only a handful of medical schools, you should still make contact and speak to the admissions tutors at those medical schools that consider retakes.

6 | Herbal medicine
Non-standard applications

So far, this book has been concerned with the 'standard' applicant: the UK resident who is studying at least two science subjects at A level/ in the IB course/Scottish Highers – and who is applying from school or who is retaking immediately after disappointing grades. However, what about students who do not have this 'standard' background, such as international students? Or those who have not studied science A levels? The main non-standard applicants and the steps they should take to apply to medical school are outlined in this chapter.

Those who have not studied science A levels

If you decide that you would like to study medicine after having already started on a combination of A levels that does not fit the subject requirements for entry to medical school, you can apply for the 'pre-medical course'.

The course covers elements of chemistry, biology and physics and lasts one academic year. It leads to the first MB qualification, for which science A levels provide exemption. If your pre-med application is rejected, you will have to spend a further two years taking science A levels at a sixth-form college. Alternatively, some colleges offer one-year A level courses, and many subjects can be covered from scratch in a single year. Check which provisions your local college has to offer. However, only very able students can cover A levels in chemistry and biology in a single year with good results. You should discuss your particular circumstances with the staff of a number of colleges in order to select the course that will prepare you to achieve the A level grades you need in the subjects you require.

Overseas students

Competition for the few places available to overseas students is fierce, and you would be wise to discuss your application informally with the medical school before submitting your UCAS application. Have a look on the universities' websites, as they publish their statistics. For example, in 2018, the University of Edinburgh had 17 international students compared to 190 UK and EU students. Many medical schools give preference to students who do not have adequate provision for training in their own countries. You should contact the medical schools individually for advice on the application procedure and costs.

Information about qualifications can be obtained from British Council offices or British embassies.

Mature students and graduates

Graduates

Course options available to graduates include the following:

- four-year graduate-entry courses
- five-/six-year courses in the normal way
- six-year pre-medical/medical courses
- Access courses.

You should check which Access courses are accepted by medical schools, as not all will consider them. Often, each medical school has a shortlist of Access courses from which it accepts applications – for example, at Keele they currently look only at Access courses from The Manchester College, College of West Anglia, Dudley College, Sussex Downs College and Stafford College. Other medical schools accept different ones. It is also usually the case that you have to reach a very high level of achievement in these courses, not just pass them.

Mature students

In recent years the options available for mature students have increased enormously. There is a growing awareness that older students often represent a 'safer' option for medical schools because they are likely to be more committed to medicine and less likely to drop out, and are able to bring to the medical world many skills and experiences that 18-year-olds sometimes lack. In general, there are two types of mature applicant:

1. those who have always wanted to study medicine but who failed to get into medical school when they applied from school in the normal way
2. those who came to the idea later on in life, often having embarked on a totally different career.

The first type of mature applicant has usually followed a degree course in a subject related to medicine and has obtained a good grade (minimum 2.i). These students have an uphill path into medicine because their early failure tends to prejudice the selectors. Nevertheless, they do not have the problem of taking science A levels at a late stage in their education. A few years ago, applicants in this position almost always had to go back to the beginning (sometimes even having to resit A levels) and then apply to the medical schools for the standard five-/six-year courses.

The second category of mature student is often of more interest to the medical school selectors and interviewers. Applications are welcomed from people who have achieved success in other careers and who can bring a breadth of experience to the medical school and to the profession.

Options available for mature students are summarised below. The chapter then examines each option in more detail.

Applicants with A levels that satisfy medical schools' standard offers

Five-/six-year courses in the normal way.

Applicants with A levels that do not satisfy standard offers

This could include arts A levels, or grades that are too low. Applicants in this category can take the following routes.

- Retake/pick up new A levels at sixth-form college.
- Enrol on a six-year pre-medical/medical course (first MBChB pre-medical entry). These are available at:
  - Cardiff
  - Dundee
  - East Anglia
  - Glasgow (one year)
  - Keele
  - King's College London
  - Lancaster (one year)
  - Leicester
  - Liverpool
  - Manchester
  - Nottingham
  - Sheffield
  - Southampton.
- These courses are usually given the code A104 by UCAS, although there are differences to this code structure. They include a foundation (pre-medical) year and are designed for students without science A level backgrounds. They should not be confused with the six-year (usually A100) courses offered by many medical schools that include an intercalated BSc. The A100 courses require science A levels.
- Enrol on an Access course (see page 169).

Mature students with no formal A level or equivalent qualifications

Applicants in this category can take the following routes:

- A levels, then five-/six-year courses in the normal way
- Access courses (see page 169).

Preparing the application

Mature students and graduates are faced with many decisions on the route to becoming a doctor. Not only do they have to decide which course or combination of courses might be suitable, but in many cases they also have to try to gauge how best to juggle the conflicting demands of study, financial practicalities and their families.

Mature students need to prepare carefully for their applications in order to ensure that they are recognised as being fully committed to a career as a doctor. As an illustration of this, take the case of Max.

Case study

Max is an architecture graduate who is now studying medicine at the University of Cambridge, having completed Biology and Chemistry A levels in one year.

'Why did I change? It was an easy one for me in the end because I simply wanted to be a doctor. What was not so simple was acknowledging that my six years' training to be an architect was something I was going to have to shelve after such an intense undertaking to get to where I was. However, I can honestly say without hesitation that I have made the right choice of route. What is more, I understand my own decision to move and that, for me is key. You need to always know why you are doing something and believe in yourself to achieve it.

'I have just finished my first term and am really enjoying it. The first couple of weeks I was quite alarmed by the intense nature of the course and the workload but it has settled down now and I am finding the intellectual rigour a positive challenge. The hardest aspect of the course is the volume of information, particularly with medicine, some sciences are quite challenging, especially with the amount you need to memorise.

'Having done A level Biology and Chemistry in a year (as I had already gone through school and done a degree), by the time I was applying I had done a lot less Chemistry than everyone else which I feel left me at a disadvantage. Due to this, my biochemistry interview was not spectacular, it was an uncomfortable interview and the interviewer was not sympathetic.'

Interviews

'My biggest enemy was stress. You have been contemplating the interview for months before you even started applying, and now, in your head, it's all or nothing. For the interview process at Cambridge, I had three interviews. There was one interview for Biochemistry, which was clinically based and another was problem solving in an applied medical context. The third interview was a mix of everything and had a fair amount of physiology.

'I then got re-interviewed at a graduate college where they are more familiar with taking people who went the same route as me. It was just one interview this time, which was a combination of all the things from the previous interviews. They started from what I had studied and went on from there rather than asking about things I had not yet covered.

'I was asked quite a few questions on why I was changing career and my motivation which were questions I welcomed. However, you could see that they were keen to press that line of questioning in order ensure that the move I was making was the right one. They also asked quite a few questions regarding the similarities between architecture and medicine, from straightforward examples to some more contextual examples.

'After my interview, I wrote down all the questions they asked and I would advise you to do the same, not so you can re-live the interview later but rather to learn from it as the one thing I have noticed is that the course has picked up where the interview left off.'

Exams

'There is no substitute for practice on the A level examinations, make sure you focus on the technique; learning and examination technique are not mutually exclusive. However, be aware, university is completely different and there is a huge gap between the two. Do not let it catch you out. My advice is to take a Pre-University course before you start so that you can bridge that gap effectively and start in the correct way.'

Tip

'The best advice I got was simply: start early. Make contact with the admissions team. I emailed asking for more and more clarification; I took any opportunity to go to meet with the admissions staff. So when the day comes for an interview, or even maybe a rejection, you can show your determination through a paper trail.'

Max's medical school interview questions were typical of those faced by not only students applying to Cambridge but also by mature students and graduates. The interviewers were interested in:

- why he had decided to change direction
- what he had done to convince himself that this was the right option for him
- what his career had given him in the way of personal qualities that were relevant to medicine
- what financial arrangements he had made to fund his studies
- whether he had found it difficult studying A levels alongside 18-year-olds
- crucially, what his scientific knowledge was like after a prolonged absence.

Case study

Rob has just started his first year at the University of Birmingham. He did a one-year intensive A level course and achieved top grades.

'I did a one year A level course as my first-choice A level subjects, despite going well, were not targeted for medicine. However, for me, this was the equivalent of a gap year and a stepping stone on the way to getting to where I wanted to go. It also gave me time to undertake some more work experience, not only for the benefit of my application but also to confirm to myself that this was the right route to follow for me.

'The course is really good at Birmingham and there is a lot of variety which ensures it is very interesting. At Birmingham you get to spend a day at a GP practice with a General Practitioner from the start, putting the things you learn into practice, which to me was a huge appeal of the course. The course is quite large, with 250 others so you get to meet a lot of people, while at the same time, there is a large emphasis on peer learning which I enjoy.

'There is a lot of context to take in and get your head around. Sometimes what you are taught at A level is a watered down version of what you will learn, so it's learning to replace that knowledge with a more accurate explanation.

'The interview process here was MMI (multiple mini interviews) and they used eight different stations. At each station there was a folder with a brief in it to read and somebody to act out a different scenario with. For example, at one station there was a role play exercise where I had to imagine the person I was speaking to was a patient who I had to tell had a high BMI which meant they were obese. This was so they can observe how you would communicate with a patient.

'However, it was difficult to gauge how the day went as you cannot read the interviewers, some of whom were really engaged and encouraging, while others were completely deadpan, which could be rather disconcerting.

'My biggest encouragement to applicants is this: research the type of course you want to do at university. I would not have been happy with a pure theory led course and I am so glad that, even though I applied for one, I am now studying an integrated course which suits and caters for my learning style.

'I think it is really important to decide that medicine is what you want to do and make sure that you are genuinely enthusiastic. Do you really want to do it? Rather than feeling you should study it or having been told by somebody else that you should study it. Try to enjoy it as there are lots of other things to do as well so don't become obsessed with the course. Remember to enjoy your time with your mates and socialise as well. The rest time for a doctor is essential to be good at your job during working time.'

Personal statement

Take your personal statement to as many sensible people who know what they are talking about as you can. Bribe teachers with coffee and chocolate. Go to science teachers for help, as the people reading the finished article tend to see things from a similar rationale; along the lines of 'Why is that there?' and 'What's the point of saying that? It's just waffle.' Keep the writing simple, make sure to write in continuous prose, don't overuse the thesaurus, and check spelling and punctuation to ridiculous extremes. Remember, spell check isn't foolproof and won't flag the difference between principle and principal, or effect and affect. It's the little things like that which could ruin a perfectly good application.

For mature applicants, the UCAS personal statement needs to be carefully structured. In most cases, insufficient space is allowed for the amount of information necessary to present a convincing case. It is usually advisable for mature applicants to send a detailed CV and covering letter direct to the medical schools once their UCAS number has been received.

For mature applicants, the personal statement should be structured as follows:

1. brief career and educational history: in note form or bullet points if necessary

2.   reasons for the change of direction
3.   what the candidate has done to investigate medicine
4.   brief details of achievements, interests, etc.: again, note form or bullet points are fine.

The most important thing to bear in mind is that you must convince the selectors that you are serious about the change in direction, and that your decision to apply to study medicine is not a spur-of-the-moment reaction to dissatisfaction with your current job or studies.

A useful exercise is to try to imagine that you are the person who will read the personal statement in order to decide whether to interview or to reject without interview. Does your personal statement contain sufficient indication of thorough research, preparation and long-term commitment? If it does not, you will be rejected. As a rough guide, at least half of it should cover your reasons for applying for a medical course and the preparation and research that you have undertaken. The further back in time you can demonstrate that you started to plan your application, the stronger it will be.

Doing a pre-medical course

Pre-medical courses or programmes are not to be confused with Access courses. As the name suggests, pre-medical courses usually act as a 'pre-medical school year' or 'year zero' before you enter medical school.

You will need to look at the website of each medical university to find out if it offers this course.

There is a pre-medical course run by Medipathways College that allows you to apply for medical school for the following year. In the event you are not successful with your medical school applications, you could progress directly into the final year of its two-year BSc, allowing you to re-apply again as a graduate. This means you would have three attempts for medical school entry.

Access courses

A number of colleges of further education offer Access to Medicine courses. The best-known and most successful of these is the course at the College of West Anglia, in King's Lynn. Primarily (but not exclusively) aimed at health professionals, the course covers biology, chemistry, physics and other medically related topics, and lasts one year. Most medical schools will accept students who have successfully completed the course. Contact details can be found at the end of the book.

Four-year graduate courses

Often known as Graduate Entry Programmes (GEPs), these are given the code A101, A102 or A109 by UCAS. These codes help you match up similar courses at different institutions and tell you which course is applicable to what you are wishing to study. The biggest change in medical school entry in recent years has been the development of these graduate-entry schemes. The first medical schools to introduce accelerated courses specifically for graduates were St George's Hospital Medical School and Leicester/Warwick (which has since split into two separate medical schools). Courses can be divided into two types:

1. those for graduates with a medically related degree
2. those that accept graduates with degrees in any discipline.

About 10% of UK medical school placements are now on GEPs. The following medical schools run GEPs, further details of which can be found on the UCAS website (in brackets is the number of places available):

- Birmingham (40)
- Cambridge (41)
- Cardiff (no quota)
- Imperial (20)
- King's (28)
- Liverpool (29)
- Newcastle (25)
- Nottingham (87)
- Oxford (30)
- Barts and the London, Queen Mary (39)
- Southampton (48)
- St George's (60)
- Swansea (75)
- Warwick (177).

The King's course differs from the others listed above, as it is also available to healthcare professionals with equivalent academic qualifications. The first year of the course is taught in London or in Kent. Students then join the other King's MBBS students for the remaining three years.

GAMSAT

Eight medical schools use the GAMSAT (Graduate Australian Medical School Admissions Test) in the UK:

- Cardiff
- Keele
- Liverpool
- Nottingham

- Plymouth or Exeter (for anyone who has not sat A levels in the last two years; healthcare professionals without a biomedical science or healthcare professional degree qualification)
- St George's
- Swansea.

Standard registrations for the GAMSAT UK test take place in early June for those sitting the test in September, and in early November for those sitting the test in March. The fee to sit the GAMSAT test is £262, but an extra charge of £60 applies if you sit the GAMSAT after the main closing date. Payment must be made by credit card at the time of completing your online registration or by bank draft after completing a provisional registration. No other payment options are available.

Candidates sit the GAMSAT examination in either March or September, and those with the best all-round scores are then called for interview. The GAMSAT examination consists of three papers:

1. reasoning in humanities and social sciences (75 multiple-choice questions) – 100 minutes
2. written communication (two essays) – 60 minutes
3. reasoning in biological and physical sciences (110 multiple-choice questions: 40% biology, 40% chemistry, 20% physics) – 170 minutes.

Private universities

At the University of Buckingham, the first private medical school in the UK started in January 2015. It costs £36,500 per year and will fast-track medical students in four-and-a-half years rather than the standard five or six years for the A100 course. The university is hoping to attract students who would otherwise have looked to study abroad.

Under the proposals set out by the Universities Minister Jo Johnson, which allow universities to raise the tuition fees if they can prove high quality teaching, there could be an increase in private institutions being given university status. The plan is to increase competition within the university sector to drive standards. This will be one to monitor over the next year or so. In 2017, Aston University admitted undergraduate medicine students for the first time, as did the University of Buckingham and the University of Central Lancashire.

Studying outside the UK

If you are unsuccessful in gaining a place at one of the UK medical schools, and do not want to follow the graduate-entry path, you might want to look at other options. Note that following the UK's decision to leave the EU, arrangements for UK students studying at institutions in other EU countries are to be negotiated as part of wider discussions with other Member States regarding the UK's exit from the EU. As those discussions are ongoing, it looks unlikely that this will have an effect on UK students studying in the EU as long as they continue to remain in the European Economic Area (EEA) generally.

One option for those who have been unsuccessful with their applications is to study medicine abroad – for example at Charles University in the Czech Republic or Comenius University in Bratislava, the capital of Slovakia. There are a number of medical schools throughout the world that will accept A level students, but the important issue is whether or not you would be able to practise in the UK upon qualification, should you wish to do so. You need to bear in mind that there is a big difference between European and non-European medical schools. In the case of medical schools based within the EU, they are usually fully recognised by the GMC under current European legislation for primary qualifications. However, one should be cautious with those based in Eastern Europe as statistics show that they often have an alarmingly high drop-out rate. They usually admit students based on a short written entrance test based in science and not always based on a traditional A level syllabus that you may have prepared for. They also do not put much emphasis on your actual A level grades, which does mean that sometimes the wrong students are admitted, which may be a factor in their high attrition rate. Please do your research and be cautious, as often it is staying in medical school that tends to be the challenge, *not* getting in.

In the EEA, in addition to the ones mentioned above, you will find examples of such medical schools as Plovdiv Medical University, Bulgaria, Masaryk University, Czech Republic, Palacky University, Czech Republic, Debrecen University, Hungary, Università degli Studi di Milano, Italy, Riga Stradins University, Latvia and Lithuania University of Health Sciences, Lithuania.

After completing a degree in the UK, students are eligible to apply for FY2 posts, though some take FY1 posts without having to sit the Professional Linguistic and Assessment Board (PLAB). Do bear in mind you will be competing with applicants who have been studying in UK medical schools up to the same point so the competition is high for internship placements.

Courses often attended by UK students include the following.

- St George's University School of Medicine in Grenada (West Indies) is the most popular and 'tried and tested' option, for those who can afford the fees. Students who wish to practise in the UK can spend part of the clinical stage of the course in a range of hospitals in the UK, including King's in London. To practise in the UK, students sit the PLAB (Professional and Linguistic

Assessments Board) test to gain limited registration; for more information, see www.gmc-uk.org/doctors/plab.asp. Clinical experience can also be gained in hospitals in the US, allowing students to practise there as well. A high proportion of the St George's University medical school teachers have worked in UK universities and medical schools.

- There are four-year medical degree courses at St Matthew's University, Grand Cayman. The first two years are taught on Grand Cayman (British West Indies) and the final two clinical years are taught in the UK or the US.
- Six-year medical degree courses are offered in Slovakia, the Czech Republic and Poland. These courses are taught in English and are recognised in the UK.
- Medical courses are taught in English at Charles University in Prague and at other universities in the Czech Republic.

In addition to the medical schools attached to UK universities, there are a number of institutions offering medical degree courses that are taught in the UK but are accredited by overseas universities – mostly based in the Caribbean, Russia or Africa. If you are considering these, you must ensure that you are fully satisfied that the courses are bona fide and that the qualification you receive will allow you to practise in the UK (or anywhere else in the world).

In order to check if your qualification is recognised in the UK, you should visit the GMC website (www.gmc-uk.org/doctors/registration_applications/acceptable_primary_medical_qualification.asp). You can also refer to the university websites, which should inform you of the validity of their degree in the UK.

Studying abroad may not be the first choice for students who were initially hoping to secure a place at home in the UK. Also, healthcare systems outside the UK are very different, so adapting to life abroad where the local language may not be English as well as studying medicine may not appeal to all.

A new alternative to five- or six-year courses abroad may be the 2+4 Articulation offered by Medipathways College in London. This allows students to complete a two-year BSc degree in London and apply (or re-apply) for a place in the UK and quite a significant number of students have been successful taking this route. However, every student is also given an optional conditional offer of a place to study medicine abroad at the start of the BSc course. This articulation allows students who would prefer to study in the UK to consider studying abroad if they have to once they have exhausted all options. This way you not only achieve a BSc in two years and get the chance to apply for a UK medical school, but you also have a secure place to study medicine abroad for just four years with friends you have already made when in London. For further information, see 'The fifth choice' section on page 25.

Getting into US medical schools

Here we can only point those who are interested in studying medicine in the US in the right direction. While it is possible for international students to study medicine in the United States, it certainly is not straightforward. Firstly, you should go to the AAMC (Association of American Medical Colleges) website at www.aamc.org. This is an excellent site, but dense. All of the member universities are listed, and by following the links most of your questions can be answered.

Furthermore, from here you can be directed to AMCAS, which is the American Medical College Application Service. For students wishing to apply, go to www.aamc.org/students/applying. The application is $160 for one application and $38 for every application thereafter. The AAMC website suggests that a very good investment is the *Medical School Admission Requirements (MSAR)* resource, which can be bought as an online resource for around $27/approximately £16.50 from https://students-residents.aamc.org/applying-medical-school/applying-medical-school-process/deciding-where-apply/medical-school-admission-requirements. Students can also apply directly to the medical schools.

Suffice it to say that the following criteria have to be met.

* You are expected to gain very high grades in A levels – nearly all straight A grades. The higher the grades, the higher your GPA (grade point average) will be; the higher your GPA, the better your chances of being selected by the more renowned universities. An A grade = 4 GPA points; a B grade = 3; and a B+ = 3.75.
* You have studied at least one year of biology, physics and English and two years of chemistry (including organic chemistry) post-16/at A level.
* You will be asked to provide two or three references from your personal tutor and teachers.
* If you are not from an English-speaking country you will be required to sit the TOEFL (Test of English as a Foreign Language). The minimum score for entry into any university is 79 out of 120. The more demanding the course (such as medicine) and the more prestigious the university, the higher this language requirement will be.
* Most universities accept the IELTS (International English Language Testing System), but it must be at 7 points or above.
* The TOEFL test can be sat in the UK.
* Fees and living costs are very high. A full list can be obtained from the AAMC website.

If you are serious about applying, you need to start as early as possible – early in the first year of your undergraduate programme is recommended. This is because you will need to research the universities as best you can, bearing in mind that the distance does not allow for quick visits to open days as for UK universities.

In the US, medicine is a postgraduate degree. All students enter the schools after doing four years of undergraduate study. In these first four years you can study something different, but you must obviously study a science-based or pre-med course. You are also expected to gain work experience in these first two years. For more information go to www.aamc.org/students/aspiring.

MCAT

Almost every medical school in the US and Canada requires students to take this examination. It is a computer-based, multiple-choice assessment, designed to test critical reasoning, problem-solving skills, writing skills and, naturally, scientific knowledge as well. It takes seven and a half hours to complete.

It comprises four sections: Chemical and Physical Foundations of Biological Systems; Biological and Biochemical Foundations of Living Systems; Psychological, Social, and Biological Foundations of Behaviour; and Critical Analysis and Reasoning Skills, with each section made up of 59 multiple-choice questions for which you have 95 minutes to answer each section. Each section is scored from 118 to 132.

This exam is to be taken in the year that you intend to start study. You can take it up to three times in a year, or four times over two years and a maximum of seven times in total in any number of years. Test dates tend to generally be in August and September each year and you are recommended to register at least 60 days beforehand to ensure that you get a space. It costs $310.

Visas

If you are studying outside the EU, you will require a visa for study. The university in question will advise you on which visa you should obtain; for example, in the USA they will advise you as to whether you require an F-1 Student or J-1 Exchange Visitor visa. You do not require a student visa for Grenada but you do require a student visa for the Cayman Islands. A good place to look first would be UKCISA (UK Council for International Student Affairs) at www.ukcisa.org.uk. Currently, while the UK remains a member of the EU, UK citizens will continue to have free movement within EU countries; arrangements for UK citizens after the UK leaves the EU are to be decided as part of the UK's exit negotiations with the other Member States.

Students with disabilities and special educational needs

If a candidate has a specific health requirement or disability there is every possibility that a medical school will be able to help. There is an area in the personal details section of the UCAS application where you can indicate the type of disability/special needs that you have. You need to select the most appropriate option from the list given. There is also a space provided for you to give any further details of the conditions that affect you.

However, each medical school has a responsibility to ensure that doctors are able to fulfil their responsibilities. The decision on fitness to practise is separate from the academic and non-academic selection process. These guidelines are set out by the GMC. You are encouraged to fully research the demands of the course before you apply to each institution. Bear in mind that in order to practise as a doctor you also have to be deemed fit to practise. The profession places huge demands on the individual and therefore you must consider all the facts from the outset.

You are equally encouraged to apply if you have a hearing or visual impairment. All institutions are fully committed to support students with special needs, from dyslexia to physical disability, and have access arrangements in place.

Once an offer is made, the medical school will contact you to discuss any appropriate arrangements that should be made. It is most likely to be the case that certain halls of residence may have physical limitations on access arrangements. It is absolutely vital that all relevant information that may impair your ability to study and potentially practise is made clear at this stage. If not, and if the issues become obvious later on in the course, it could possibly result in the candidate being withdrawn from the course.

In terms of special educational needs, students who require a word processor or extra time will be allowed these in the same way that they would have been at school, subject to providing the correct documentation to the university.

For more information refer directly to the university.

Some useful websites

Access-Ability: www.accessability-uk.com
Hope for Disabled Doctors: www.hope4medics.co.uk

7 | Prevention rather than cure
Fees and funding

To find out the fees and funding for medical courses, prospective students should explore each of the universities' websites and/or talk to the universities' financial departments. This is because fees and funding procedures vary from university to university. Factors affecting the fees and overall debt can include:

- where the student is from
- geographic (does the student live in a city?)
- the amount of help that parents can give
- if the student receives a scholarship
- whether the student has found work.

Whatever the circumstances, a student must give serious consideration to the cost and be prepared to fully commit. Your choice also has to involve careful financial planning for the four or five years that a course may last. On top of the tuition fees, you will have to consider living costs; needless to say, in big cities such as London, living costs will be much higher than in other parts of the country. One estimate is that London will cost about £10,555 per year to cover food, accommodation, travel and books.

Fees

UK students

In the past 12 months an important piece of law for students was enacted. The Higher Education and Research Act 2017 allows universities to charge UK and EU students up to £9,250 a year for tuition fees (for those institutions offering high quality education) as part of the government's new Teaching Excellence Framework (TEF). While there was also talk of another wave of tuition fees changes, at the Conservative Party conference in October 2017, the government opted to freeze tuition fees, not yet taking the cost over £9,500. The TEF will assess participating universities and colleges on the quality of their teaching. The higher-ranked universities will be able to charge the maximum amount, £9,250, though they are not unanimous in terms of when and whether they will effect this. Tuition fee loans will also increase to cover the higher fees. The fee cap for students studying in Wales remains at £9,000, while fees for students starting courses in Northern Ireland are £9,250, unless you are a student from Northern Ireland or the EU, in which case the fee is less.

Scottish universities charge the now standard £1,820 for all Scottish and EU students; fees are paid by the SAAS, subject to residence requirements. Students from England, Wales and Northern Ireland pay up to £9,250. In Northern Ireland, the fee for EU students and those from Northern Ireland is £4,160 and the fee for all other UK students is up to £9,250.

You should refer to the websites of the specific universities to find out what they intend to charge, and also to the UCAS website, using the course search facility.

If you are a student resident in England you will pay up to £9,000 if you study in Wales, and up to £9,250 in the rest of the UK.

If you are a student resident in Scotland you will pay a set £1,820 tuition fee if you study at a Scottish university, with the Student Awards Agency for Scotland (SAAS) paying those fees if you meet eligibility criteria. You will pay up to £9,000 if you study in Wales and up to £9,250 in England and Northern Ireland.

If you are a student resident in Wales you will pay up to £9,000 if you study in Wales, and up to £9,250 if you study in the rest of the UK. However, you will be able to receive a £4,296 loan from the Welsh Government (£4,046 if studying in Wales), and you will also be eligible for a grant up to the difference between the loan and the full fee.

If you are a student resident in Northern Ireland you will pay up to £9,000 if you study in Wales and up to £9,250 if you study in England or Scotland, but you will pay only up to £4,160 if you study in Northern Ireland. Students from Northern Ireland will be able to apply for a tuition fee loan to cover all or part of the fees; the amount you receive will vary depending on which country you choose to study in.

EU students

If you are an EU student you will pay up to £9,250 if you study in England, but there is no fee if you study in Scotland as the SAAS will pay the tuition fees for you if you are EU domiciled and meet the eligibility requirements. If you study in Wales you will pay up to £9,000 and receive the same help as Welsh students (see above) subject to the current terms. If you study in Northern Ireland, you will pay up to £4,160.

Implications of Brexit

With Britain voting to leave the European Union, many universities were concerned about what that would mean for European student numbers at each institution. There will be no fee implications for students for 2017 entry; EU students starting their course in September 2017 will pay home fees for the duration of their course. More importantly, EU students starting their courses in September 2017 remain eligible to apply for student funding under the current terms. This was confirmed by Jo Johnson, Minister for Universities and Science, in September 2016.

On 11 October 2017, the government announced that EU students applying to study in the UK will be eligible for the same grants and loans as domestic students, and for now will continue to pay the same fees as home students.

Table 11 Tuition fees by region for courses starting in 2018

Student's home region	Location of university or college			
	England	Scotland	Wales	Northern Ireland
England	Up to £9,250	Up to £9,250	Up to £9,000	Up to £9,250
Scotland	Up to £9,250	No fee	Up to £9,000	Up to £9,250
Wales	Up to £9,250	Up to £9,250	Up to £9,000	Up to £9,250
Northern Ireland	Up to £9,250	Up to £9,250	Up to £9,000	Up to £4,160
EU	Up to £9,250	No fee	Up to £9,000	Up to £4,160
Non-EU	Variable	Variable	Variable	Variable

International students

Home students – that is, UK nationals – and, currently, EU students pay lower tuition fees than non-EU/UK students. For international students from outside these two regions, the costs can be prohibitive. The fees for non-EU international students do not have a set upper limit – they will depend on the course and the university. For example, in 2018 the University of Dundee was charging students £32,000 per year of study. The Scottish Government has also introduced a mandatory levy for international students of £10,000 per year in order to cover the cost of NHS clinical teaching.

In the past few academic years the tuition fees charged to non-EU students were typically between £14,000 and £19,000 per year for the pre-clinical courses and between £21,000 and £39,000 per year for the clinical courses.

This can be even higher; for example, for 2018 entry, Imperial College will charge a flat rate of £40,000 per year for international students for both clinical and non-clinical courses. This amounts to £240,000 in total, a change from the consistent approach of recent years. This will remain the case, barring inflationary increases, for the foreseeable future.

Nevertheless, whether you are a UK/EU resident or an international student, the truth of the matter is that, unless you are wealthy, the usual scenario is that you will accumulate a large debt.

Funding: bursaries and grants

Currently, universities charging more than £6,000 must provide financial support for students from disadvantaged backgrounds, though this may change in light of the recent fee increases. You can find out more at:

- www.ucas.com/ucas/undergraduate/undergraduate-student-finance-and-support
- www.gov.uk/student-finance.

As a result of the tuition fees increases, though it will differ from university to university, in general each institution will provide income support of roughly maximum £3,000 dependent on family household income.

If you live in England, there is no longer a maintenance grant to cover your living costs. Instead, all money available to students for living expenses will be provided as a maintenance loan, to be paid back once students start earning £21,000 or more. Figures for students from different parts of the UK will vary slightly. For further details please refer to the UCAS website, www.ucas.com. You may be entitled to other grants and bursaries; for details of how to find more information, see page 182.

Changes to funding

According to the Royal Medical Benevolent Fund (www.rmbf.org/medical-students), the following is accurate with regard to funding.

- Students will not pay tuition fees before they start or while they are studying a course.
- You may apply for a student loan, which is partially income-assessed.
- There have been increases in the Disabled Students' Allowance.
- There have been major changes to income assessment for new and continuing students from Scotland.

NHS bursary

Currently, students studying for medical degrees recognised by the General Medical Council may be eligible for financial assistance from the NHS for part of their course. The arrangements vary depending on your country of residence, and are set out briefly below. Note: While the rules have changed for new students in some health-related fields from 1 August 2017, provision for medicine students has not been amended in the new guidelines.

Students in England will have their tuition fees paid by the NHS Student Bursary scheme from their fifth year of study onwards. They will also be able to apply for a means-tested NHS bursary for living costs, as well as a reduced maintenance loan dependent on where you live from Student Finance England. The bursary award also includes access to a non-means tested grant of £1,000. This funding information is also applicable to graduate students from their fifth year of study.

Students in Wales can apply for a means-tested NHS Bursary (administered by Students Awards Services) from the fifth year of their course, as well as a reduced student loan. In 2017/18 they would also receive a non-means tested grant of £1,000 and a maintenance loan of up to £3,392. Graduate students on accelerated four-year programmes will be eligible for NHS funding from their second year of study onwards.

Students in Northern Ireland are eligible for income-assessed bursaries from their fifth year onwards. The bursaries are administered by the Department of Health, and tuition fees are also paid by the Department for the duration of the bursary. While in receipt of the bursary, students can also apply for a reduced maintenance loan from Student Finance Northern Ireland.

Tuition fees for Scottish students studying in Scotland are paid by the Student Awards Agency Scotland (SAAS) for the duration of the course. Students can apply to the SAAS for maintenance support, which includes loans and bursaries and do not have any changes in their funding from their fifth year of study.

Further details and guidelines are available on the NHS Health Careers website at www.healthcareers.nhs.uk/i-am/considering-or-university/financial-support-university/financial-support-medical-and-dental.

Student loans

The most common way in which students are able to fund themselves is by taking out a student loan, of which there are two types: a loan for fees and a loan for living costs. As of October 2017, in a shifting of policy, the government announced that students will start repaying these loans only once they have finished studying and are earning over £25,000 for students in England and Wales, and over £17,775 for students in Scotland and Northern Ireland, with repayments made at incremental steps based on earnings. Most universities can put you in touch with loan agencies and with the NHS.

How to apply for financial support: UK students

New students in England

- Ask for an application form from the local authority (LA) in whose area you normally live.
- Ask for an application form from the Student Loan Company (SLC).
- Apply online or download a form (form PN1) from the gov.uk website (www.gov.uk/student-finance-forms).

New students in Northern Ireland

- Ask for an application form from the Education and Library Board (ELB) in whose area you normally live.
- Apply online or download a form (form PN1) from the Student Finance Northern Ireland website (www.studentfinanceni.co.uk).

New students in Wales

- Apply to the LA in whose area you normally live.
- Apply online or download a form (form PN1) from the Student Finance Wales website (www.studentfinancewales.co.uk).

New students in Scotland

- Apply to the Student Awards Agency for Scotland (SAAS) wherever you live in Scotland.
- Apply online or download a form (form SAS3) from the SAAS website (www.saas.gov.uk).

Other sources of funding for medical students

There are various websites that will give you information on a variety of organisations that can offer scholarships, grants and bursaries that are available in addition to the NHS bursary. These include the following.

- **Access Agreement bursaries:** non-repayable bursaries, though because each individual university decides, it is not possible to give an estimate of their worth (except in Scotland, where a fee waiver or bursary scheme may be an alternative for students from Scotland).
- **Armed forces bursaries/cadetships:** these are generous and may be worth considering, provided you are happy to commit to an agreed number of years working as a doctor in the Army, Navy or Air Force.
- **Medical awards and competitions:** these are of varying amounts and varying levels of competitiveness.

- **University bursaries:** many universities often provide bursaries for low-income students. If your household income is below £17,910 you will probably receive a bursary. Some universities give bursaries to people with higher incomes. It is worth investigating this with your university.
- **Hardship loans:** if you are having financial problems you can apply for additional sources of funding from your institution; roughly up to £500 can be added to your current student loan.

For more information on these, go to www.medschoolsonline.co.uk and www.gov.uk/student-finance/extra-help.

Scholarships and prizes

There are also many scholarships and prizes that are run by the many professional medical organisations. Some of the applications may require a supporting statement from a member of academic staff. Check the criteria carefully before applying.

- **British Association of Dermatologists:** offers two lots of £3,000 towards fees and living expenses for an intercalated-year project related to dermatology and skin biology. It also offers nine lots of £500 as undergraduate project grants and three lots of £250 essay prizes.
- **Sir John Ellis Student Prizes:** students submit a description of a piece of work, survey, research or innovation in which they have been directly involved in the field of medical education. First prize in each category is £300 plus expenses (conference fee, accommodation in halls of residence, annual dinner and standard travel expenses). Runners-up will have the conference fee and accommodation in the halls of residence paid for.
- **The Genetics Society Summer Studentship scheme:** this provides funding for undergraduate students to spend their summer vacation working in a genetics laboratory in order to gain research experience: £200 for up to eight weeks and £750 to contribute for costs incurred in the lab work. There are different grants available to cover any course-specific costs.
- **The Nuffield Foundation:** a scheme similar to the Genetics Society Summer Studentship is also run by the Nuffield Foundation.
- **The Physiological Society:** the Society offers grants for students undertaking research of a physiologic nature under the supervision of a member of the society during a summer vacation or intercalated BSc year (if the student is not receiving LA or other government support).
- **The Pathological Society:** funding is offered for students wanting to intercalate a BSc in pathology who do not have LA or other government support. The Society also offers awards to fund electives and vacation studies in pathology.

- **The Junior Association for the Study of Medical Education (JASME) Essay Prize for Medical Education:** the Association offers a £100 first prize and a £50 runner-up prize.

Fees for studying abroad

You should not expect the same level of financial support if you want to study overseas. Currently, you have the right as a UK citizen to pay the same fees in another EU country as nationals of that country; you can find out more about financial support on the Your Europe website at www.europa.eu/youreurope/citizens. There are a few grants and scholarships available through UK charities, and these are listed on the UKCISA (www.ukcisa.org.uk) and UNESCO (www.unesco.org.uk) websites.

8 | The doctor will see you now
Careers in medicine

This chapter looks briefly at some of the possible careers open to prospective medics. It is of value to have an idea and indeed some understanding of the possibilities and avenues open to you both while you are studying and for the interview. Arguably some knowledge here could be of great benefit if you are asked questions such as 'Have you given any thought to future prospects?' or 'Where do you see yourself in 10 years?' at interview.

The paths and avenues open to members of the medical profession once they graduate are too numerous to go into in detail here. As a trainee doctor nearing the end of your study, questions such as the prospect and possibility of specialisation and about where you might like to work have to be answered. The best advice we can give here is to make sure to research as much as possible, talk to people and, above all, be aware of the areas in medicine that you have enjoyed the most.

Apart from specialisations (see below), there is a wide range of areas that doctors may end up working in. Obviously, most people understand that many doctors become GPs. However, there are also as many who dedicate their lives to working in the state-funded NHS. Within the NHS there is a panoply of possibilities, such as working in public health, working in medical management and administration and even working in research.

Away from public hospitals, there are careers to be made in private enterprise, for example running a consultancy business such as plastic surgery. Some doctors opt for the armed forces and others work for the police as forensic psychiatrists and forensic pathologists. Another area is education, in terms of lecturing, research and writing while working for a university. It is not uncommon to find doctors who have a portfolio of work, spending some of their time in hospitals, doing private consultancy in their own surgeries and teaching or doing research. Such a life is not only well remunerated but also stimulating.

First job

The training programme for doctors called Modernising Medical Careers (MMC) became fully functional in 2007. The training is part of the

Certificate of Completion of Training (CCT). Before the MMC, newly qualified doctors would spend a year at Pre-registration House Officer level, dividing the period between medicine and surgery. After that, the junior doctor would be working as a Senior House Officer (SHO) for a number of years before applying for a Specialist Registrar post.

MMC is summarised in Figure 3 (see below).

In the last year of the medical degree, medical students apply for a place on the Foundation programme. The Foundation programme is designed to provide structured postgraduate training on the job and lasts two years. The job starts a few weeks after graduation from medical school. In the first few weeks there might be a short period of 'shadowing', to help new doctors get used to the job. After successful completion of the first year, they will gain registration with the GMC.

The Foundation programme job is divided into three four-month posts in the first year. These posts will typically consist of:

- four months of surgery (e.g. urology, general surgery)
- four months of another specialty (e.g. psychiatry, GP)
- four months in a medical specialty (e.g. respiratory, geriatrics).

The second year is again divided into three four-month posts, but here the focus is perhaps on a specialty or may include other jobs in shortage areas.

Final year at medical school: apply for a place on a two-year Foundation programme (www.foundationprogramme.nhs.uk)

↓

Foundation programme starts in August
F1: three four-month placements (medicine, surgery, specialty)
F2: three four-month placements (some choice of placements)
During F2, apply for specialty registrar training (SpR) or GP registrar training

↓

Specialty training begins
SpR: five to seven years
GP registrar: approximately three years
After completion, receive Certificate of Completion of Training (CCT) and be eligible to go onto the SpR or GP Register

↓

Apply for senior posts, e.g. consultant

Figure 3 MMC training structure

There is talk of whether to remove the provisional registration of newly qualified doctors, meaning that after completion of the MBBS degree, students will be fully registered with the GMC. This would not remove the need for the Foundation years' training, however, as these are still critical for developing a doctor's knowledge and skills. This has not yet been approved; however, it is the case that you cannot be provisionally registered for any longer than three years and 30 days (1125 days).

For more information on the application procedure, visit:

- www.medschoolsonline.co.uk/index.php?pageid=157
- www.foundationprogramme.nhs.uk

Specialisations

The MMC was introduced in 2005. It aims to provide information to doctors applying for specialty training within the NHS in England. It provides details on how to apply and the changes that occur to the recruitment and the application process. In 2012, for the first time, an agreed standardised timetable was produced for all applicants by all of the UK health departments.

Specialist training programmes typically last for five to seven years. After gaining the CCT, a doctor is then eligible to apply for a Certificate of Eligibility for Specialist Registration (CESR). Either will make you eligible for entry to the GMC's Specialist Register or GP Register.

To do this you will need to apply for postgraduate medical training programmes in the UK to the deanery or 'unit of application' directly. In this application process you will be competing for places on specialty training programmes with other doctors at similar levels of competence and experience.

For more information, visit the MMC website at http://specialtytraining. hee.nhs.uk.

Here follow the 10 major specialisations available in medicine, each with its own sub-specialisations and some selected elaborations:

1. accident and emergency
2. anaesthetics
3. general practice
4. intensive care
5. medical specialties
   o cardiovascular disease
   o clinical genetics
   o clinical pharmacology and therapeutics
   o dermatology
   o endocrinology and diabetes mellitus
   o gastroenterology
   o general medicine

- o genito-urinary medicine
- o geriatrics
- o infectious diseases
- o medical oncology
- o nephrology (renal medicine)
- o neurology
- o occupational medicine
- o paediatrics
- o palliative medicine
- o rehabilitation medicine
- o rheumatology
- o tropical medicine
6. obstetrics and gynaecology
7. pathology
   - o bacteriology
   - o blood transfusion
   - o chemical pathology
   - o diagnostic radiology
   - o forensic pathology
   - o haematology
   - o histopathology
   - o immunology
   - o medical microbiology
   - o neuropathology
   - o radiology
   - o radiology and nuclear medicine
   - o radiotherapy
8. psychiatry
   - o adult psychiatry
   - o child and adolescent psychiatry
   - o forensic psychiatry
   - o old age psychiatry
   - o psychiatry of learning difficulties
9. public health medicine
   - o clinical public health
   - o government medical service
   - o medical administration
10. surgical specialties
    - o general surgery
    - o neurosurgery
    - o ophthalmology
    - o otolaryngology
    - o paediatric surgery
    - o plastic surgery
    - o thoracic surgery
    - o urology.

A few selected specialisations, briefly described, follow.

Anaesthetist

An anaesthetist is a medical doctor trained to administer anaesthesia and manage the medical care of patients before, during and after surgery. Anaesthetists are the single largest group of hospital doctors and their skills are used throughout the hospital in patient care. They have a medical background to deal with many emergency situations.

They are also trained to deal with breathing, resuscitation of the heart and lungs and advanced life support.

Audiologist

Audiologists identify and assess hearing and/or balance disorders, and from this will recommend and provide appropriate rehabilitation for the patient. The main areas of work are paediatrics, adult assessment and rehabilitation, special needs groups and research and development.

Cardiologist

This is the branch of medicine that deals with disorders of the heart and blood vessels. These specialists deal with the diagnosis and treatment of heart defects, heart failure and valvular heart disease.

Dermatologist

There are over 2,000 recognised diseases of the skin but about 20 of these account for 90% of the workload. Dermatologists are specialist physicians who diagnose and treat diseases of the skin, hair and nails such as severe acne in teenagers, which happens to be a very common reason for referral. Inflammatory skin diseases such as eczema and psoriasis are very common and without treatment can produce significant disability.

Emergency

Often referred to as the type of medicine practised in accident and emergency departments. It requires doctors to be dynamic and ready to adapt and respond at a moment's notice. Departments are led by consultants but rely on teamwork to help patients who are in an urgent condition. As you might be required to make life-saving decisions in a pressurised situation you will need a lot of confidence and belief to be in this role.

Gastroenterologist

A gastroenterologist is a medically qualified specialist who has sub-specialised in the diseases of the digestive system, which include ailments affecting all organs, from mouth to anus, along the alimentary canal. In all, a gastroenterologist undergoes a minimum of 13 years of formal classroom education and practical training before becoming a certified gastroenterologist.

General practitioner (GP)

A GP is a medical practitioner who specialises in family medicine and primary care. They are often referred to as family doctors and work in consultation clinics based in the local community.

GPs can work on their own or in a group practice with other doctors and healthcare providers. A GP treats acute and chronic illnesses and provides care and health education for all ages. They are called GPs because they look after a whole person, and this includes their mental health and physical well-being.

Gynaecologist

Gynaecologists have a broad base of knowledge and can vary their professional focus on different disorders and diseases of the female reproductive system. This includes preventive care, prenatal care and detection of sexually transmitted diseases, smear-test screening and family planning. They may choose to specialise in different areas, such as acute and chronic medical conditions, for example cervical cancer, infertility, urinary tract disorders and pregnancy and delivery.

Immunologist

Immunologists are responsible for investigating the functions of the body's immune system. They help to treat diseases such as AIDS/HIV, allergies (e.g. asthma, hay fever) and leukaemia using complex and sophisticated molecular techniques. They deal with the understanding of the processes and effects of inappropriate stimulation that are associated with allergies and transplant rejection, and may be heavily involved with research. An immunologist works within clinical and academic settings as well as with industrial research. Their role involves measuring components of the immune system, including cells, antibodies and other proteins. They develop new therapies, which involves looking at how to improve methods for treating different conditions.

Neurologist

A neurologist is a medical doctor who has trained in the diagnosis and treatment of nervous-system disorders, which includes diseases of the brain, spinal cord, nerves and muscles. Neurologists perform medical examinations of the nerves of the head and neck, muscle strength and movement, balance, ambulation and reflexes, memory, speech, language and other cognitive abilities.

Obstetrician

These are specialised doctors who deal with problems that arise during maternity care, treating any complications that develop in pregnancy and childbirth and any that arise after the birth. Some obstetricians may specialise in a particular aspect of maternity care such as maternal medicine, which involves looking after the mother's health; labour care, which involves care during the birth; and/or foetal medicine, which involves looking after the health of the unborn baby.

Paediatrician

This is a physician who deals with the growth, development and health of children from birth to adolescence. To become paediatricians, doctors must complete six years of extra training after they finish their medical training. There are general paediatricians and specialist paediatricians such as paediatric cardiologists. They work in private practices or hospitals.

Plastic surgeon

Plastic surgery is the medical and cosmetic specialty that involves the correction of form and function. There are two main types of plastic surgery: cosmetic and reconstructive.

1. Cosmetic surgery procedures alter a part of the body that the person is not satisfied with, such as breast implants or fat removal.
2. Reconstructive plastic surgery involves correcting physical birth defects, such as cleft palates, or defects that occur as a result of disease treatments, such as breast reconstruction after a mastectomy, or from accidents, such as third-degree burns after a fire.

Plastic surgery includes a variety of fields such as hand surgery, burn surgery, microsurgery and paediatric surgery.

Psychiatrist

Psychiatrists are trained in the medical, psychological and social components of mental, emotional and behavioural disorders. They specialise in the prevention, diagnosis and treatment of mental, addictive and emotional disorders such as anxiety, depression, psychosis, substance abuse and developmental disabilities. They prescribe medications, practise psychotherapy and help patients and their families cope with stress and crises. Psychiatrists often consult with primary care physicians, psychotherapists, psychologists and social workers.

Surgeon

A general surgeon is a physician who has been educated and trained in diagnosis, operative and post-operative treatment, and management of patient care. Surgery requires extensive knowledge of anatomy, emergency and intensive care, nutrition, pathology, shock and resuscitation, and wound healing. Surgeons may practise in specific fields such as general surgery, orthopaedic, neurological or vascular and many more.

Urologist

A urologist is a physician who has specialised knowledge and skills regarding problems of the male and female urinary tracts and the male reproductive organs. Extensive knowledge of internal medicine, paediatrics, gynaecology and other specialties is required by the urologist.

Some alternative careers

Armed forces

Doctors in the army are also officers, and provide medical care for soldiers and their families (www.gov.uk/government/organisations/ministry-of-defence/about/recruitment).

Aviation medicine (also aerospace medicine)

The main role is to assess the fitness to fly of pilots, cabin crew and infirm passengers (for further information go to the website of the Faculty Occupational Medicine www.fom.ac.uk).

Clinical forensic medical examiner (police surgeon)

Clinical forensic physicians or medical examiners spend much of their time examining people who have been arrested. Detainees either ask to see a doctor or need to be examined to see if they are fit for interview or fit to be detained (www.csofs.org).

Coroner

The coroner is responsible for inquiring into violent, sudden and unexpected, unnatural or suspicious deaths. Few are doctors, but some have qualifications in both medicine and law (see the section on clinical forensic and legal medicine on The Royal Society of Medicine website at www.rsm.ac.uk).

Pathologist

This job requires a variety of different specialisms, all of which combine to help form the basis of medical diagnosis. Whether it be chemical pathology, haematology, histopathology or immunology, each of which then breaks down further, there is a variety of opportunities available in clinical and lab-based research work.

Pharmaceutical medicine

Job opportunities for doctors in pharmaceutical medicine include clinical research, medical advisory positions and becoming the medical director of a company. Patient contact is limited but still possible in the clinical trials area (www.abpi.org.uk).

Prison medicine

A prison medical officer provides healthcare, usually in the form of GP clinics, to prison inmates (www.crglocums.uk.com).

Public health practitioner

Public health medicine is a specialty that deals with health at the level of a general population rather than at the level of the individual. The role can vary from responding to outbreaks of disease that need a rapid response, such as food poisoning, to the long-term planning of health-care (www.fph.org.uk).

> 'What is special about Medicine? Everything and nothing. Everything because you have the ability to help and make a difference to people's lives. Nothing, because once you go into this career, it is your duty and part of your every day routine. What you do matters but it is also expected. You must be serious about what you want to do because there will be many relying on you. It is tremendously rewarding and that is why anyone should go to work. In regards to the application, simply be true to you; that is the best starting place.'
>
> *Dr Emma Lumley*

9 | An apple a day
Further information

Courses

Students often have a variety of reasons for wanting to dedicate their professional lives to medicine. However, each aspiring 'future doctor' must ensure that this career choice has been an informed one. In essence, panels look for each applicant to be able to map out the next 14 years of their lives, identifying what skills they would need to develop at each step of the career ladder in order to achieve their goal of expertise in a specialty of their choice. The slow and steady progression provides a career that is often both physically and mentally demanding yet fulfilling, as the doctor's input into the multidisciplinary team results in better patient care.

It is impossible to get a true idea of what medicine entails from just attending a course or talking to careers advisers. However, there are some organisations that aim to help students gain a realistic impression of medicine as a whole. Medsim is one such organisation.

Medsim specialises in helping students in their preparation for the highly competitive medical school application process by offering both patient contact and practicals. It hosts short courses at the University of Nottingham which are designed to fit a lot of work experience into a short space of time in order to give students a full picture of the work doctors have to do and this includes: Case Histories, Surgical Techniques for Keyhole Surgeries, Patient Rounds, Keyhole Surgery and Suturing. These clinical and surgical skills will both benefit a student's UCAS application and cost as little as £199 for a two-day residential course. See https://medlink-uk.net/medsim to find out more.

There is also an *OnTrak* virtual course that Medlink runs to go through all aspects of the UCAS application and UKCAT examination, and others. For more information go to https://medlink-uk.net/wp-content/uploads/2014/07/Ontrak.pdf.

Publications

Careers in medicine

A Career in Medicine: Do You Have What it Takes? (2nd edition), ed. Rameen Shakur, Royal Society of Medicine Press

The Insider's Guide to UK Medical Schools, eds Sally Girgis, Leigh Bisset, David Burke, BMJ Books

Learning Medicine: How to Become and Remain a Good Doctor, Peter Richards, Simon Stockill, Rosalind Foster, Elizabeth Ingall, Cambridge University Press

Genetics

The Blind Watchmaker, Richard Dawkins, Penguin

Genome, Matt Ridley, Fourth Estate

The Language of the Genes, Steve Jones, Flamingo

Who's Afraid of Human Cloning? Gregory E. Pence, Rowman and Littlefield

Y: The Descent of Man, Steve Jones, Abacus

Higher education entry

HEAP 2019: University Degree Course Offers, Trotman Education

Getting into Oxford & Cambridge: 2019 Entry, Trotman Education

How to Complete Your UCAS Application: 2019 Entry, Trotman Education

Preparing for the BMAT, Heinemann

Medical science: general

Asimov's New Guide to Science, Isaac Asimov, Penguin

Aspirin: The Extraordinary Story of a Wonder Drug, Diarmuid Jeffreys, Bloomsbury

Don't Die Young, Dr Alice Roberts, Bloomsbury

Everything You Need to Know About Bird Flu and What You Can Do to Prepare For It, Jo Revill, Rodale

The Greatest Benefit to Mankind: A Medical History of Humanity, Roy Porter, Fontana

The Human Brain: A Guided Tour, Susan Greenfield, Phoenix

Human Instinct, Robert Winston, Bantam

The Noonday Demon: An Anatomy of Depression, Andrew Solomon, Vintage

Pain: The Science of Suffering (Maps of the Mind), Patrick Wall, Weidenfeld and Nicolson

Penicillin Man: Alexander Fleming and the Antibiotic Revolution, Kevin Brown, History Press

From Poison Arrows to Prozac: How Deadly Toxins Changed Our Lives Forever, Stanley Feldman, John Blake Publishing

A Short History of Nearly Everything, Bill Bryson, Black Swan

A User's Guide to the Brain, John Ratey, Abacus

Medical ethics

The Body Hunters: Testing New Drugs on the World's Poorest Patients, Sonia Shah, The New Press

Causing Death and Saving Lives: The Moral Problems of Abortion, Infanticide, Suicide, Euthanasia, Capital Punishment, War and Other Life-or-death Choices, Jonathan Glover, Penguin

Medical practice

Bedside Stories: Confessions of a Junior Doctor, Michael Foxton, Atlantic Books

NHS Plc: The Privatisation of Our Health Care, Allyson M. Pollock, Verso

Websites

All the medical schools have their own websites (see below) and there are numerous useful and interesting medical sites. These can be found using search engines. Particularly informative sites include the following.

- Admissions forum: www.newmediamedicine.com (essential information for applicants)
- BMAT: www.admissionstestingservice.org/for-test-takers/bmat/about-bmat
- BMA: www.bma.org.uk
- Department of Health: www.dh.gov.uk
- GMC: www.gmc-uk.org
- Student BMJ: student.bmj.com
- UKCAT: www.ukcat.ac.uk
- WHO: www.who.int

Financial advice

For information on the financial side of five to six years at medical school, see www.money4medstudents.org. This website has been prepared by the Royal Medical Benevolent Fund, in partnership with the BMA Medical Students Committee, the Council of Heads of Medical Schools and the National Association of Student Money Advisers.

Examiners' reports

The examining boards provide detailed reports on recent exam papers, including mark schemes and specimen answers. Schools are sent these every year by the boards. They are useful when analysing your performance in tests and mock examinations. If your school does not have copies, they can be obtained from the boards themselves. The examining boards' website addresses are:

- www.aqa.org.uk
- http://qualifications.pearson.com
- www.ocr.org.uk
- www.wjec.co.uk.

Contact details

Studying in the UK

Aberdeen
The School of Medicine, Medical Sciences and Nutrition
University of Aberdeen
3rd Floor Polwarth Building
Foresterhill
Aberdeen AB25 2ZD
Tel: 01224 437923
Email: medadm@abdn.ac.uk
Web: www.abdn.ac.uk/study/courses/undergraduate/medicine/medicine

Barts and The London School of Medicine and Dentistry
Garrod Building
Turner Street
London E1 2AD
Tel: 020 7882 8478
Email: smdadmissions@qmul.ac.uk
Web: www.smd.qmul.ac.uk

Birmingham
College of Medical and Dental Sciences
University of Birmingham
Edgbaston
Birmingham B15 2TT
Tel: 0121 414 3858
Email: mdsenquiries@contacts.bham.ac.uk
Web: www.medicine.bham.ac.uk

Brighton and Sussex Medical School
BSMS Teaching Building
University of Sussex
Brighton BN1 9PX
Tel: 01273 643528
Email: medadmissions@bsms.ac.uk
Web: www.bsms.ac.uk

Bristol
Faculty of Medicine and Dentistry
First Floor South
Senate House
Tyndall Avenue
Bristol BS8 1TH
Tel: 0117 394 1642
Medical and dentistry admissions coordinator: Mrs J.L. Bennett
Email: med-admissions@bristol.ac.uk/jo.bennett@bristol.ac.uk
Web: www.bris.ac.uk/medical-school

Buckingham Medical School
The University of Buckingham
Hunter Street
Buckingham
MK18 1EG
Tel: 01280 827546
Email: medicine-admissions@buckingham.ac.uk
Web: medvle.buckingham.ac.uk

Cambridge
University of Cambridge
School of Clinical Medicine
Box 111 Cambridge Biomedical Campus
Cambridge CB2 0SP
Tel: 01223 333308
Email: admissions@cam.ac.uk
Web: www.medschl.cam.ac.uk

Cardiff
Institute of Medical Education
Cardiff University School of Medicine
Cochrane Medical Education Centre
Heath Park
Cardiff CF14 4YU
Tel: 029 2068 8113/8101, ext. 88101
Email: medadmissions@cardiff.ac.uk/deanmeded@cardiff.ac.uk
Web: www.medicine.cf.ac.uk

Dundee
Ninewells Hospital and Medical School
Dundee DD1 9SY
Tel: 01382 383838
Email: asrs-medicine@dundee.ac.uk
Web: www.medicine.dundee.ac.uk

East Anglia
Medical Admissions
Norwich Medical School
Faculty of Medicine and Health Sciences
University of East Anglia
Norwich NR4 7TJ
Tel: 01603 591515
Email: enquiries@uea.ac.uk
Web: www.uea.ac.uk/med

Edinburgh
Edinburgh Undergraduate Admissions
College of Medicine and Veterinary Medicine
The Chancellor's Building
49 Little France Crescent
Edinburgh EH16 4SB
Tel: 0131 650 1000
Email: medug@ed.ac.uk
Web: www.ed.ac.uk/schools-departments/medicine-vet-medicine

Exeter
School of Medicine
University of Exeter
St Luke's Campus
Heavitree Road
Exeter EX1 2LU
Tel: 01392 725500
Email: ug-ad@exeter.ac.uk
Web: http://medicine.exeter.ac.uk

Glasgow
College of Medical, Veterinary and Life Sciences
Wolfson Medical School Building
University of Glasgow
University Avenue
Glasgow G12 8QQ
Tel: 0141 330 6216
Email: med-sch-admissions@glasgow.ac.uk
Web: www.gla.ac.uk/colleges/mvls

Hull York
Hull York Medical School
John Hughlings Jackson Building
University of York
Heslington
York YO10 5DD
Tel: 01904 321782 (admissions)
Email: admissions@hyms.ac.uk
Web: www.hyms.ac.uk

Imperial College London
Imperial College
Level 2, Faculty Building
South Kensington Campus
London SW7 2AZ
Tel: 020 7594 7259
Email: medicine.ug.admissions@imperial.ac.uk
Web: www.ic.ac.uk/medicine

Keele
School of Medicine
David Weatherall Building
Keele University
Staffordshire ST5 5BG
Tel: 01782 733937
Email: medicine@keele.ac.uk
Web: www.keele.ac.uk/medicine

King's College London
Faculty of Life Sciences and Medicine
King's College London
1st Floor, Henriette Raphael Building
Guy's Campus
London SE1 1UL
Tel: 020 7848 7890
Email: ug-healthadmissions@kcl.ac.uk
Web: www.kcl.ac.uk/medicine

Lancaster
Lancaster Medical School
Lancaster University
Lancaster LA1 4YW
Tel: 01524 594547
Email: medicine@lancaster.ac.uk
Web: www.lancaster.ac.uk/lms

Leeds
The Admissions Section
School of Medicine
Room 7.09, Level 7
Worsley Building
University of Leeds
Leeds LS2 9JT
Tel: 0113 343 4379
Email: ugmadmissions@leeds.ac.uk
Web: www.leeds.ac.uk/medhealth

Leicester
University of Leicester Medical School
Centre for Medicine
Lancaster Road
Leicester LE1 7HA
Tel: 0116 252 2969/2985
Email: med-admis@le.ac.uk
Web: www2.le.ac.uk/departments/msce/undergraduate/medicine

Liverpool
School of Medicine
University of Liverpool
Cedar House
Ashton Street
Liverpool L69 3GE
Tel: 0151 795 4370
Web: www.liverpool.ac.uk/medicine

Manchester
The Medical School
Faculty of Medical and Human Sciences
University of Manchester
Oxford Road
Manchester M13 9PL
Tel: 0161 306 0211
Email: ug.medicine@manchester.ac.uk
Web: www.medicine.manchester.ac.uk

Newcastle
Administrator for Admissions
Medical Student Office
School of Medical Education
University of Newcastle
Newcastle upon Tyne NE2 4HH
Tel: 0191 222 7005
Email: medic.ugadmin@ncl.ac.uk
Web: www.ncl.ac.uk/biomedicine

Nottingham
Medical School
Faculty of Medicine and Health Sciences
University of Nottingham
Queen's Medical Centre
Nottingham NG7 2UH
5- and 6-year Medicine (A100 & A108) Tel: 0115 951 5559
4-year Graduate Entry Medicine (A101) and BSc Medical Physiology
and Therapeutics Tel: 01332 724900
Email: medschool@nottingham.ac.uk
Web: www.nottingham.ac.uk/mhs

Oxford
Medical Sciences Divisional Officer
University of Oxford
Level 3, John Radcliffe Hospital
Oxford OX3 9DU
Tel: 01865 285783
Email: admissions@medschool.ox.ac.uk
Web: www.medsci.ox.ac.uk

Plymouth
Peninsula College of Medicine and Dentistry
John Bull Building
Tanmer Science Park
Research Way
Plymouth PL6 8BU
Tel: 01752 437333
Email: meddent-admissions@plymouth.ac.uk
Web: www.plymouth.ac.uk/schools/peninsula-school-of-medicine

Queen's Belfast
School of Medicine, Dentistry and Biomedical Sciences
Whitla Medical Building
97 Lisburn Road
Belfast BT9 7BL
Tel: 028 9097 2215
Email: pjmedschool@qub.ac.uk
Web: www.qub.ac.uk/schools/mdbs

St Andrews
School of Medicine
University of St Andrews
Medical and Biological Sciences Building
North Haugh
St Andrews KY16 9TF
Tel: 01334 461886
Email: admissions@st-andrews.ac.uk; medicine@st-and.ac.uk
Web: http://medicine.st-andrews.ac.uk

St George's
University of London
Cranmer Terrace
London SW17 0RE
Tel: 020 8672 9944
Email: study@sgul.ac.uk
Web: www.sgul.ac.uk

Sheffield
The Medical School
University of Sheffield
Beech Hill Road
Sheffield S10 2RX
Tel: 0114 222 5531
Email: medadmissions@sheffield.ac.uk
Web: www.shef.ac.uk/medicine

Southampton
Faculty of Medicine
University of Southampton
Southampton General Hospital
Building 85
Life Sciences Building
Highfield Campus
Southampton SO17 1BJ
Tel: 023 8059 4408
Email: ugapply.fm@southampton.ac.uk
Web: www.southampton.ac.uk/medicine

Swansea
College of Medicine
Grove Building
University of Wales Swansea
Singleton Park
Swansea SA2 8PP
Tel: 01792 513400
Email: medicine@swansea.ac.uk
Web: www.swan.ac.uk/medicine

UCL (and Royal Free)
UCL Medical School
University College London
74 Huntley Street
London WC1E 6BT
Tel: 020 7679 0841
Email: medicaladmissions@ucl.ac.uk
Web: www.ucl.ac.uk/medicalschool

Warwick
Warwick Medical School
University of Warwick
Coventry CV4 7AL
Tel: 02476 574880
Email: wmsinfo@warwick.ac.uk
Web: www2.warwick.ac.uk/fac/med
Note: Warwick is a graduate-entry only university, not A level entry.

Access to Medicine
The College of West Anglia
Tennyson Avenue
King's Lynn PE30 2QW
Tel: 01553 761144
Email: enquiries@cwa.ac.uk
Web: www.cwa.ac.uk

Studying outside the UK

Royal College of Surgeons in Ireland
123 St Stephen's Green
Dublin 2
Ireland
Tel: +353 1 402 2248 or 2156
Email: admissions@rcsi.ie
Web: www.rcsi.ie

Saint George's University School of Medicine
University Centre
Grenada
West Indies
Admission Advisor: Angela McCabe
Tel: 0800 169 9061 ext. 9 1380 (from the UK)
Tel: +1 (631) 655 8500 ext. 1328
Email: sguenrolment@sgu.edu
Web: www.sgu.edu

Volunteering

Positive East
(HIV/AIDS volunteering)
159 Mile End Road
London E1 4AQ
Tel: 020 7791 2855
Email: volunteering@positiveeast.org.uk
Web: www.positiveeast.org.uk

vInspired
5th floor, Dean Bradley House
52 Horseferry Road
London SW1P 2AF
020 7960 7000
Email: info@vinspired.com
Web: https://vinspired.com

NHS Choices
Web: www.nhs.uk/livewell/volunteering/Pages/Volunteeringhome.aspx
Web: www.medicalcareers.nhs.uk/considering_medicine/work_
experience/volunteering.aspx

British Red Cross
British Red Cross
UK Office
44 Moorfields
London EC2Y 9AL
Tel: 0344 871 1111
Email: information@redcross.org.uk
Web: www.redcross.org.uk/Get-involved/Volunteer

Do-it (database for volunteering placements)
Web: www.do-it.org.uk

Community Service Volunteers (CSV)
Volunteering Matters
The Levy Centre
18–24 Lower Clapton Road
London E5 0PD
Tel: 020 7278 6601
Web: https://volunteeringmatters.org.uk

Working Abroad
Web: www.workingabroad.com/volunteer-organisations
Web: www.gapmedics.co.uk

It is worthwhile also contacting your local county or borough council to find out what volunteering opportunities it has, for example, in care homes or schools (both of which will require criminal record DBS checks).

Tables

Table 12 Medical school admissions policies for 2018–19

Institution	Usual offer	Usual A level requirements	Retakes considered
Aberdeen	AAA (IB 36 points with 3 at HL, Grade 6)	None	Yes, but advice should be taken from previous interview and extenuating circumstances evidence submitted
Aston	AAB	Biology or Chemistry	Yes on a case by case review
Barts and The London	AAA	Two must be sciences, either Biology or Chemistry, no Further Mathematics	Only with serious extenuating circumstances under the Equalities Act
Birmingham	A*AA (IB 32 points, with HL 7,6,6)	Biology and Chemistry	No
Brighton and Sussex	AAA (IB 36 points, with 6, 6 in Biology and Chemistry)	Biology + Chemistry at A grades	In extenuating circumstances and if narrowly missed by one grade
Bristol	AAA (IB 36 points with 18 points at HL)	Chemistry at A grade + 1 other lab-based science (one of Human Biology, Biology or Physics)	In extenuating circumstances
Buckingham	AAB (IB 36 points, with 6, 6 in Biology and Chemistry)	Chemistry and at least one other science or Maths subject; achieved in one sitting	-
Cambridge	A*A*A (IB 40–42 with HL 7,7,6)	Chemistry + 2 other science/Maths	In extenuating circumstances
Cardiff	AAA (IB 36 with 19 at HL inc. 7, 6, 6)	Biology/Chemistry	If previously applied to Cardiff
Dundee	AAA (IB 37 inc. 6 in HL Chemistry and another science)	Chemistry + 1 other science/Maths	No
East Anglia A100	AAA (IB 36 inc. 6 in all HL subjects)	Biology	Yes (ABB or A*A*C from first sitting)
East Anglia A104	BBB	No usual requirements	No

Table 12 Continued

Institution	Usual offer	Usual A level requirements	Retakes considered
Edinburgh	AAA (IB 37, with HL 6,6,7)	Chemistry + 1 other science/Maths + B in GCSE English; only one of Maths and Further Maths	In extenuating circumstances (evidence must be verified prior to UCAS application)
Exeter	A*AA–AAA (IB36–38)	Chemistry + Biology/Physics	Yes (AAB at first attempt, then A*AA/AAA)
Glasgow[1]	AAA (IB 38, with 6 in HL Biology and Chemistry and Mathematics or Physics)	Chemistry + 1 other science/Maths + B in GCSE English	No
Hull York	AAA (IB 36,with HL 6,6,5)	Biology + Chemistry at grade As	In extenuating circumstances
Imperial	A*AA (IB 38, with 6 in HL Biology and Chemistry)	Chemistry and/or Biology or one science subject and Maths	In extenuating circumstances and if previously applied to Imperial (CCC at first sitting and AAA in retake examinations and it is mentioned in referee's statement)
Keele	A*AA–AAA (IB 35, with 6 in all HL subjects)	Biology/Chemistry + another science	No
King's	AAA (IB 35 inc. 7, 6, 6 in Biology and Chemistry)	Biology/Chemistry	In extenuating circumstances
Lancaster	AAAb–A*AA (IB 36 inc. 6 in Biology and Chemistry)	Biology + Chemistry, only one of Maths or Further Maths	Will consider applicants who have taken longer than two years
Leeds	AAA (IB 35, with 6 in HL Chemistry plus 2 other subjects)	Chemistry at grade A	In extenuating circumstances
Leicester	AAA (IB 36 inc. 6 in all subjects)	Chemistry	In extenuating circumstances and if previously held Leicester offer
Liverpool	AAA (IB 36. with 6 in HL Biology and Chemistry)	Biology, Human Biology + Chemistry + 3rd + 4th AS	In extenuating circumstances (minimum CCC at first attempt)
Manchester	AAA (IB 37, with HL 7,6,6)	Chemistry + 1 other science	In extenuating circumstances and if narrowly missed AAA; reapplications encouraged
Newcastle	AAA (IB 38 inc. 6 in Biology and Chemistry)	Biology/Chemistry	In extenuating circumstances with supporting evidence from GP or school

Table 12 Continued

Institution	Usual offer	Usual A level requirements	Retakes considered
Nottingham	AAA (IB 36, with 6 in HL subjects)	Biology, Human Biology, + Chemistry	In extenuating circumstances
Oxford[2]	A*AA (IB 39, with HL 7, 6, 6)	Chemistry + Biology and/or Physics and/or Maths	See advice on website
Plymouth	A*AA–AAA (IB 36–38)	Chemistry + Biology/Physics	Yes (AAB at first attempt then A*AA/AAA)
Queen's Belfast	AAAa (IB 36, with 6 in HL subjects)	Chemistry + Biology/Physics	If previously held Queen's offer and missed by 1 grade (AABa at first attempt)
St Andrews	AAA (IB 38, with HL 6,6 and 6)	Chemistry + 1 other science/Maths, need to be predicted A*AA	In extenuating circumstances
St George's	AAA (IB 36, with 18 points and 6 in Biology and Chemistry)	Biology/Chemistry	No
Sheffield	AAA (IB 36, with 6 in HL subjects and no less than 4 in all SL subjects)	AAA in Chemistry + other science	No
Southampton	AAAa (IB 36, with 6 in HL subjects)	Biology/Chemistry	In extenuating circumstances and if retaking one subject
UCL	A*AA (IB 39, with 19 in HL subjects with 6 in every course)	A* in either Biology or Chemistry	Not recommended to apply

[1] Retake candidates will normally be expected to achieve AAA.
[2] Oxford offers two courses:

* A100: a six-year course in medicine (graduates may apply and complete this course in five years). Contact address: Administrative Officer, Medical Sciences Teaching Centre, South Parks Road, Oxford OX1 3PL; tel: 01865 285783; email: admissions@medschool.ox.ac.uk

* A101: a four-year accelerated course (for graduates in applied or experimental sciences). Contact address: Medical Sciences Office, John Radcliffe Hospital, Headington, Oxford OX3 9DU; tel: 01865 228975; email: Lesley.maitland@medsci.ox.ac.uk

Note: Details were correct when going to press – check websites for updated information.

Table 13 Medical school interview and written test policies for 2017–18

Institution	Typical length (minutes)	Number on the panel	Test	Typical UKCAT score boundary (offers made 2016/17)
Aberdeen	MMI: 60, 7–9 stations × 7	–	UKCAT	1,660–2,480
Barts and The London	15–20	2–3	UKCAT	1,720–2,620 (Situational Judgement Band used)
Birmingham	MMI: 42, 7 interviews × 6	–	UKCAT	
Brighton and Sussex	MMI: 54, 5 stations × 10	–	BMAT	
Bristol	MMI: 60, multiple stations	–	UKCAT	
Cambridge	2 × 20–30 though some MMI interviews of 9 × 5 mins are being introduced	2–3	BMAT	
Cardiff	MMI: 10 stations x 6	–	UKCAT	No minimum threshold
Dundee	MMI: 10 stations × 7	–	UKCAT	Average was 2,740 for those receiving offers
East Anglia	MMI: 50, 7 stations × 5	–	UKCAT: case history discussion	No minimum
Edinburgh	Undergraduates not normally interviewed	–	UKCAT	All scores considered
Exeter	MMI: 21, 7 stations x 3	2–3	UKCAT	Overall UKCAT score considered
Glasgow	15–20, 2 panels	2	UKCAT	900–2,700
Hull York	45, Group interview and 2 personal interviews	7	UKCAT	Over 2,000 approx. Situational Judgement Band 4 not applicable
Imperial	15 for undergraduate	5	BMAT	
	15 for postgraduate	3–4	BMAT	
Keele	MMI: 45, 9 stations × 5	–	UKCAT	Excludes those in bottom 20%

Table 13 Continued

Institution	Typical length (minutes)	Number on the panel	Test	Typical UKCAT score boundary (offers made 2016/17)
King's	MMI: 45	–	UKCAT	Average 630–735 in 2015
Lancaster	MMI: 12–14 stations × 5	–	BMAT	
Leeds	MMI: 8 stations × 7	–	BMAT	
Leicester	MMI: 8 stations	–	UKCAT	UKCAT mark scored out of 24 (see website)
Liverpool	MMI: 12 stations x 5	–	UKCAT	2,500 or more
Manchester	MMI: 7 stations	3	UKCAT	c. 2,810
Newcastle	MMI		UKCAT	c. 2,473
Nottingham	MMI: 60, 8 stations x 5	–	UKCAT	Excludes bottom 50%
Oxford	2 × 20–30	2–4	BMAT	
Plymouth	20	2–3	UKCAT	Overall UKCAT score considered 2,610 in 2015/16
Queen's Belfast	MMI: 45, 9 stations × 5	–	UKCAT	Banding before interview
St Andrews	MMI: 6 stations	2–3	UKCAT	900–2,700
St George's	MMI: 40, 8 stations × 5	–	UKCAT	2,600
Sheffield	MMI: 8 stations × 8	3	UKCAT	1,850–2,700
Southampton	Selection day – an interview and a group task	2	UKCAT	2,500
UCL	15–20	2–3	BMAT	
Warwick	Graduate Entry, MMI	–	UKCAT	Those with the highest UKCAT scores were considered for interview – 2,800

MMIs are multiple mini interviews, a series of small interviews or tasks the candidate has to complete. Their content varies with the medical school that carries them out. See the individual websites for more details.
Source: University websites; correct at going to print.

Glossary of terms

AIDS (acquired immune deficiency syndrome)
AIDS is a disease that affects the immune system, lowering the body's resistance to infection. The disease is caused by the human immuno-deficiency virus (HIV).

BHA (British Humanist Association)
The association acting for those who are non-religious who seek to live ethical lives on the basis of reason and humanity.

BMA (British Medical Association)
The professional medical association and trade union for doctors and medical students.

BMAT (BioMedical Admissions Test)
An admissions test required by certain universities. See Table 5 on page 49 for a list of universities that require this test.

BMI (body mass index)
Indicates whether someone is overweight or underweight, based on their weight and height.

CBL (Case-based learning)
The medical training that some medical schools use that is more case led, based on clinical examples, than the more problem-based learning courses.

CSP (Chartered Society of Physiotherapists)
Professional, educational and trade union body for the UK's physiother-apy workforce.

GAMSAT (Graduate Australian Medical School Admissions Test)
A test introduced in 1999 by some universities to aid in the selection of candidates who already have degrees.

GEP (Graduate Entry Programme)
A four-year programme offered by universities for students who already have a degree, as opposed to the traditional five-year programme.

GMC (General Medical Council)
The governing body that protects, promotes and maintains the health and safety of the public by ensuring proper standards in the practice of medicine.

H5N1
An influenza subtype, also known as avian flu or 'bird flu'.

Integrated courses
Those where basic medical sciences are taught concurrently with clinical studies. Thus, this style is a compromise between a traditional course and a PBL course.

Intercalated degree
An intercalated degree is a one-year course of study after the preclinical years to attain a further degree, e.g. in biochemistry or anatomy.

MB (Bachelor of Medicine)
One of the three degrees that can be awarded by medical schools to students after four or five years of academic study.

MBBS (Bachelor of Medicine and Surgery)
One of the three degrees that can be awarded by medical schools to students after four or five years of academic study.

MBChB
Some medical schools award this degree instead of the MBBS. This depends on the medical school.

MMC (Modernising Medical Careers)
An association within the NHS that provides doctors with information on specialist training.

MMR (measles, mumps and rubella)
A vaccination given to young children around the age of one.

MRI (magnetic resonance imaging)
A medical imaging technique used in radiology to visualise detailed internal structures of the body.

MRSA (methicillin-resistant *Staphylococcus aureus*)
A bacterium responsible for several difficult-to-treat infections in humans. It is also called multidrug-resistant bacteria.

NICE (National Institute for Health and Clinical Excellence)
NICE sets standards for quality healthcare and produces guidance on medicines, treatments and procedures.

PBL (problem-based learning)
The medical training that some medical schools use and is a more patient-oriented approach than the more traditional lecture styles.

Personal statement
The written document provided by the candidate about themselves which is sent with the university application to the medical schools.

PLAB
The Professional Linguistic and Assessment Board is a test for assessing eligibility for students entering the UK to practise medicine having studied abroad.

SARS (severe acute respiratory syndrome)
A very serious form of pneumonia which saw an outbreak in 2002 and 2003.

Student BMJ
A publication produced for prospective medical students.

Traditional courses
Longer established and following a lecture-based style, using didactic methods. The majority of these courses are subject-based ones, where lectures are the most appropriate way of delivering the information.

UCAS (Universities and Colleges Admissions Service)
The central body through which students apply to medical school or any higher education college.

UCAS codes
The identifying letters and numbers of the various university courses. These are vital when making your application. Medical courses range from A100 to A104 depending on previous experience (e.g. A levels, degree, etc.).

UKCAT (United Kingdom Clinical Aptitude Test)
An application test that certain medical schools require students to sit before accepting them onto the course. See Table 4 on page 36 for a list of which universities require this test.

WHO (World Health Organization)
A specialised agency of the United Nations that acts as a coordinating authority on international public health.

Work experience
Voluntary work (normally) organised before you apply to medical school which is described in your personal statement. This is a vital component of your application.

Postscript

If you have any comments or questions arising from this book, the staff of MPW would be very happy to answer them. You can contact us at the address given below. Good luck with your application to medical school!

James Barton and Simon Horner

MPW (London)
90/92 Queen's Gate
London SW7 5AB
Tel: 020 7835 1355
Fax: 020 7259 2705
Email: enquiries@mpw.ac.uk